AJN

American Journal of Nursing

The Leading Voice of Nursing Since 1900

Reflections
on Nursing

80 *inspiring stories on the*
art and science of nursing

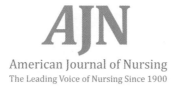

AJN

American Journal of Nursing

The Leading Voice of Nursing Since 1900

Reflections on Nursing

80 *inspiring stories on the*
art and science of nursing

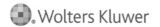

Philadelphia • Baltimore • New York • London
Buenos Aires • Hong Kong • Sydney • Tokyo

Acquisitions Editor: Nicole Dernoski
Product Development Editor: Maria M. McAvey
Production Project Manager: Priscilla Crater
Creative Director: Larry Pezzato
Manufacturing Coordinator: Kathleen Brown
Marketing Manager: Linda Wetmore
Prepress Vendor: SPi Global

Library of Congress Cataloging-in-Publication Data
Title: American journal of nursing : reflections on nursing : 80 inspiring stories on the art and science of nursing.
Other titles: American journal of nursing (Wolters Kluwer) | American journal of nursing.
Description: Philadelphia : Wolters Kluwer, [2017] | Reprints of the Reflections columns from the American journal of nursing. | Includes index.
Identifiers: LCCN 2016038504 | ISBN 9781496359063
Subjects: | MESH: Nursing | Philosophy, Nursing | Nurse's Role—psychology | United States | Collected Works
Classification: LCC RT82 | NLM WY 16 AA1 | DDC 610.73092/2—dc23 LC record available at https://lccn.loc.gov/2016038504

Preface

A Note to the Reader

In 1983, the *American Journal of Nursing* debuted *Reflections*, a column devoted to narrative writing about memorable experiences. The short essays are authored mostly by nurses, but also by other health care professionals, patients and family members, and others who have a story to tell. Readers have told us that they often turn to this section first when they take up each new issue. It's always rated as one of the journal's most popular sections.

Why does *Reflections* resonate so deeply with readers? Perhaps it's because nursing is a stressful occupation requiring considerable knowledge of biological and social sciences, critical thinking in a fast-paced environment, and often, the performance of invasive procedures on patients whose illnesses may have rendered them anxious and fearful. Narrative essays allow for introspection and reflection on the meaning of what has transpired. They are, as well, a way of bearing witness to the varieties of human suffering and possibility.

Many *Reflections* columns relate experiences that have left indelible imprints on the writer—a death that should not have occurred, a questionable course of action, an unforgettable encounter, a fractured relationship. But there are also many uplifting essays that detail the triumphs of providing care, teaching someone to be self-sufficient, achieving a new self-understanding, resolving discord, or perhaps seeing a loved one experience peaceful death. The one thing all the essays have in common is a good story that engages the reader.

This collection offers up a sampling of the articles we've published over the years. We hope you enjoy them.

Maureen Shawn Kennedy, MA, RN, FAAN
Editor in Chief,
American Journal of Nursing

Reflections on Nursing

80 *inspiring stories on the art and science of nursing*

Career Is a Forking Path

Connecting/Disconnecting

Lessons Learned

Getting Started

All in the Family

Doctor Jekyll and Doctor Hyde

From the Other Side

Memorable Patients

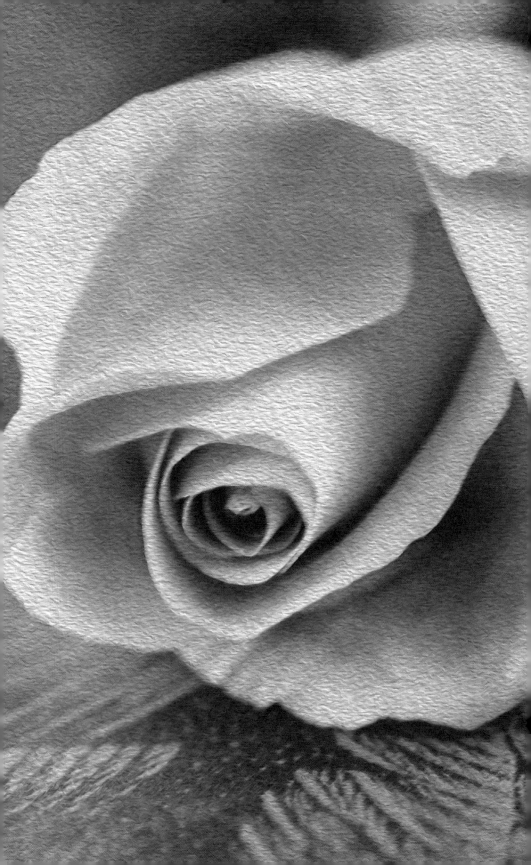

Heartbreakers

Stories of great loss witnessed or experienced—pediatric tragedies, hospice stories, hard choices about treatment or the end of life.

"I stood in the doorway and watched a family subtract a member right before my eyes."

Amanda L. Richmond, BSN, RN-BC

The Grief Train

There's no lesson plan for recovering from loss.

Cheryl A. Dellasega, PhD, RN, CRNP

As an assistant professor on tenure track, I was assigned to teach Death and Dying, an elective course. Although I had worked clinically with many grieving people and experienced personal losses, the daunting syllabus covered everything from the history of death rituals to euthanasia.

After a harrowing first semester, it got easier to teach the course. Surprisingly, in a small auditorium packed with over 100 upperclassmen, students were always willing to share tender feelings. They spoke of near-death experiences, the slow demise of a beloved family member or friend, personal recovery from serious illness, drive-by shootings and other forms of violence, abortion, suicide attempts, and traumatic accidents they blamed themselves for. Often, there were tears, and sometimes, referrals to counseling.

Always, there was a search for better answers than mine:

"How do you know people *ever* finish grieving?"

"What exactly makes it harder to live without a child than a parent?"

Eventually, another junior faculty was assigned to teach Death and Dying, and I went on to join a study that required focus groups about end-of-life care. The issues that emerged there were strikingly similar to those voiced by my students.

Then came "the Morning." There was coffee, the newspaper, and ironed shirts. I was getting ready for a student's dissertation defense and Paul, my husband, faced his own challenging day. As I prepared to shower, a crash sounded beyond the bedroom door. Something about the silence that followed made me grab my robe and go running.

My middle-aged husband was sprawled at the bottom of our basement steps, as peaceful as a young boy floating down a stream on a hot summer afternoon, arms and legs loose and eyes closed. I was able to keep his heart and breath going until the ambulance crew arrived.

Months earlier, an older married couple we loved died within months of each other. He had Parkinson's and she had cancer; it was painful to witness their mutual decline. After one visit, Paul shook his head and said, "Don't let that happen to me. Just pull the plug and give me morphine."

In the ED, when a physician showed me a CT scan outlining the flood of blood in my husband's brain, I wondered if the declaration had been some kind of morbid déjà vu.

The ventilator was turned off and the nurses administered morphine, even though they assured me he wasn't in pain. Family and friends waited until his heart rhythm dwindled to nothing and his breathing slowed, then quit.

In the months that followed, I was tunned by my failure to manage any aspect of grief. Sleep became my preferred activity of daily living because in the light stages of slumber, Paul's voice would seem to rumble in the next room, or stairs would squeak under his step. Three times he appeared in dreams, so much like his living self that I awoke in the midst of a conversation with him.

For months, I could only eat nutrition bars that tasted like cardboard. I lost so much weight I was referred to an eating disorder specialist, who diagnosed the anorexia of grief.

As the first anniversary of Paul's death approached, I booked a cross-country train trip. It wasn't to meet new people or see new scenery, but a desperate attempt to grab onto something bigger than my life.

I slept, showered, and ate on board, all new experiences. Passing through the Midwest, I took my laptop into the clear-domed observation car, intending to write about my sorrows but sightseeing instead. The next morning, I woke to the Columbia River Gorge in Oregon, a place too beautiful to be captured by a cell phone camera focused through a train window.

Everywhere, there were metaphors for life and loss—homeless people squatting in the Sacramento station during morning rush hour, "family style meals" eaten with strangers, and memories of other train trips, with and without Paul. As we headed back east, I still didn't believe the pain of loss would ever go away.

That's when a woman in the compartment across from mine struck up a conversation. As we crossed miles of Mississippi water and swampland, our stories spilled out. She was older, but also a nurse and a recent widow.

"We had a wonderful and long life together. He survived his cancer for more years than anyone thought he could, so I'm grateful," she said with a slow nod. Hours later when she got off the train, a shimmer of her peace remained.

Late that night, the long, low train whistle reminded passengers that someone was guiding us safely forward while we slept. Guru Elisabeth Kübler-Ross's stages of grieving kept time with the wheels rocking against the track as I drifted into dreams: "denial," "anger," "bargaining," "depression," and finally, "acceptance."

No amount of expertise could have prepared me for such a sudden and searing loss. My students had pressed me for better, more specific answers, but as my train sped onward, I understood just how few there really were. ▼

The Hardest Decision

Summoned from overseas, a husband and father finds a drastically altered future.

Amanda L. Richmond, BSN, RN-BC

That she was still beautiful made her situation all the more tragic. She had little visible damage. An EVD tube snaked out from under her hair and deposited its contents into a drip chamber. Her chest rose and fell at a preselected rate of 14 breaths per minute. iv lines disappeared under her gown and terminated into a central line. On the monitor, her vital signs were flawless.

Her outward appearance did nothing to suggest the chaos lying under her skull. A passenger in a vehicle that had flipped multiple times at highway speed, she'd suffered a severe traumatic brain injury. She was the only person injured out of the five involved. In the near future, the other four would come to visit her and find themselves racked with guilt while they thanked God that they'd been spared. She had two young children, a three-year-old and a newborn, as well as a military husband who was stationed overseas.

He arrived in the middle of the night, still in military regalia. His hand trembled when he shook mine. He was dry-eyed, but I could see the muscles bunching in his jaw. He followed me into his wife's room. "She doesn't look that bad," he said, with hope in his voice.

I quietly explained her injuries to him.

We spoke about her care and condition and then I retreated to give him some privacy. He sat in the chair I had placed next to her bed and took her hand. I could see his shoulders shaking and I knew he was grieving for her— and for himself and their children as well. I could see his lips moving, but I don't know if he was pleading to God or to her, begging for her life back.

He stayed for a couple of hours, and I silently wove myself around him to tend to her various lines. When he finally stood to leave, he said, "Call me when she wakes up." I didn't have the heart to remind him that she wouldn't. Instead I just told him I would call if there were any changes.

When I arrived at work the next evening, he had again taken up his vigil at her side. This time he had a crying baby with him. Noticing the tension and frustration in his face, I went in to see if I could help out. He angrily thrust the baby at me. "My own son doesn't even know me," he said. "I've been gone since before he was born."

I wrapped the baby up like a little burrito and jiggled him gently as I paced the room. In a little while, he stopped crying. Silently praying that he wouldn't start up again, I handed him back to his father, who tentatively folded him into his arms.

Looking at his wife, he said, "I can't do this by myself. I need you to wake up and help me." His voice was almost shrill, and I could see he was on the edge of losing it. I sat down next to him and he started talking. He shared stories about her and their life together. As he talked, he cried, and I funneled tissues to him until he ran out of tears. When the hiccuping finished, and the last deep breath was gone, he looked at me sheepishly, then down at his baby, who'd slept through it all. I patted his shoulder and left.

The next few nights passed uneventfully. He would often bring their two children in. On one occasion the three-year-old pointed to the ventilator and said, "Daddy, what's that?"

"That's mommy's TV," he replied, "and it's playing a really boring show."

He struggled daily to make the correct decisions for her. Would we fit her with a tracheostomy and a feeding tube or would he withdraw care and say goodbye? He had no idea how to proceed. On the fifth night by her side, he asked me what I would do. Of course, I couldn't tell him. Instead, I challenged him to consider what she would want, to make decisions based on her needs, not his own.

The following night he made the decision to withdraw care. We asked everyone—her parents, two children, and husband—to step out as we removed the tubes and lines sustaining the patient. Then we invited the family back in to spend the remaining time with her. With everything removed, she was back to being the beautiful young woman she had always been, if only for a short time. Her breaths got farther and farther apart until there were no more. I stood in the doorway and watched a family subtract a member right before my eyes.

Her husband was the last to leave the room. As he did, he hugged me tightly and said his wife would have thanked me too if she could have. I was amazed and humbled that in his grief he would think of my feelings. ▼

The Price of a Miracle

A nurse and a partner—when neither role is clear.

V. Jude Forbes, MSN, FNP

My phone rings at 4:30 AM but stops before I can pick up. It's too early for anything but bad news. Caller ID displays the number and name of a local hospital. I try to convince myself that it was a wrong number and return to sleep. What are the odds? If Dave had been admitted to the hospital, the caller wouldn't have hung up. I phone the hospital and ask for Mr. Cameron's nurse. Yes, a voice confirms, a Mr. Cameron has been admitted with chest pain. Dave apparently tried to call me from triage.

I drop to my knees to ask for strength. I prepare a pot of coffee. I hop into the shower. The routine has become all too familiar. In the car, I try to convince myself that it wasn't a heart attack. From what I've been told, the nerves on transplanted hearts have been removed, so transplantees don't experience the pain of ischemia.

When I arrive, Dave is hooked up to two IV drips, a telemeter, and oxygen as two technicians await his approval for a bedside chest X-ray and echocardiogram. He is angry and demanding to leave against medical advice. And I snap, telling him that since he called me from the ED at 4:30 AM, by God, he'd better stay until they rule out any problems. Then I ask the medical staff about enzymes, strips, troponin.

More than six years after Dave's transplantation, I still have to deal with the "let's withhold information" game, as physicians and nurses try to figure out the relationship between the old, bald white guy with the tattoos and goatee and this much younger, chunky black woman. Even though in Dave's wallet and on his paperwork I'm listed as his partner and his next of kin and given medical power of attorney, more than once I'm asked whether I'm his sitter or an LPN. Hell, my name is permanently etched on his body, along with the names of his mother, siblings, and our daughter. But I don't point this out. I simply inform them, again and again, it seems, that I'm his partner and I'm also in a postmaster's nurse practitioner program.

Dave undergoes his third angioplasty and second stent in a year. The diagnosis for the early-morning chest pain was 99% occlusion of the left anterior descending branch of the left coronary artery. But no heart attack. The cardiologist tells me that the surgery was successful, that perfusion to his heart is excellent. He says he wouldn't be surprised if Dave has five or more years in him.

Four days later the situation suddenly changes. His prognosis goes from five years to 12 hours. If that. Dave's cardiologist is visibly shaken. He says that Dave has experienced spontaneous stent closure. It sounds like he's talking to me through water. When he explains that this occurs in fewer than 3% of patients who've undergone percutaneous transluminal coronary angioplasty, the roar in my head grows louder. From his lips come the words "massive infarct." I can't take this. I interrupt him. I ask whether Dave is alive or dead. I can't integrate any of this information until I know whether we are talking about the living or the dead.

About four years after transplantation, Dave shared with me that he sometimes regretted it. This made me ashamed of him; I was offended, angry. How could someone regret life? Didn't he know how hard we all worked? Didn't he realize that he was a member of a very small group of miracle patients? How dare he regret the sacrifice the donor family made? How could he question the gift that allowed him to have more years with our daughter?

Years later, sitting in yet another coronary care unit, I finally understood that he hadn't been expressing a lack of gratitude. Instead, he realized that miracles come at a price. After transplantation, he was unable to return to work. Along with "post-pump syndrome" (a complication of being on the heart–lung machine, resulting, in Dave's case, in confusion, memory loss, and other cognitive deficits) and the adverse effects of the medications, he battled severe depression, developed significant physical debility, and had been forced to file for bankruptcy.

The heart attack was severe. Dave's on a dopamine drip and a balloon pump. I bring in a copy of his advance directives.

But Dave survives the first 12 hours. Then the next, and the next. Within 72 hours, his heart is beating on its own.

He awakens angry, confused, combative. He spits on the nurses and tries to pull out his tubes. He spews epithets and nearly breaks one nurse's hand. He's put in four-point restraints. My newest battle is to convince the staff that this isn't his mental baseline. This is not "my Dave." To anyone who will listen, I explain that even though he looks like an old Harley-riding wrestling star, Dave drives a Geo Prism, wears trifocals, has a lap cat named Daisy, and is the parent support for our daughter's after-school girls' empowerment group. I bring the nurses Krispy Kreme donuts.

I'm detaching. So is our daughter, Sloane. She doesn't ask about her dad. Her dad, when lucid, doesn't ask about her. And I'm sinking. Why didn't we ever marry? What joy have we had since the transplantation? What progress have we made as a couple? I walk into the room and say, "I know you hate everyone, but you still love me, right?" He looks up, lips slightly upturned, his pale blue eyes boring into me. "I really fucking hate you." Everyone on the unit stops as his words ring out. I'm as alone as I've ever been.

On the fifth day of hospitalization, Dave is taken out of restraints. He wakes up only to raise hell. But the man who is combative and confused shocks everyone when he sets up his medications flawlessly.

I'm torn between being a partner and being a nurse. Ultimately, I opt for being a nurse. I have more success when I treat Dave as a patient: the structure and familiarity of nursing practice are reliable. Now I side with the nurses; he is the "patient from hell."(How could I convince them otherwise after what he said to me?) In all honesty, I really hate him.

If they had asked me when Dave was admitted whether he would ever want aggressive measures to be taken—such as a balloon pump, a dopamine drip, and several days of conscious sedation, when the previous hours had featured emergency angio-plasty, insertion of a stent, closing of a stent, and a massive anterior wall infarct—I would have said no. Now he was alive because I had not been asked to make such a decision.

A week after discharge, Dave looks 10 years younger. He has dropped about 20 lbs., has more energy, and is clearer, mentally, than I've seen in years. He is driving. He spends almost every waking hour engaged in some activity. He has almost completely redecorated the house and dusted all of its bric-a-brac. He's performing acts of kindness unlike any I've seen him perform before. He donated an old computer to a neighbor and a television and PlayStation to a local teen recreation center. The man who has left Texas only once in the past decade has suddenly decided to visit his family in Wisconsin. Dave, Sloane, and I are planning our first trip—ever. He is happy.

But Dave's new life has left me without grounding, like an untethered kite. ▼

No Regrets

There is such a thing as a good death.

Arlene Koch, RN

Ray Troyan was curled in the fetal position, rocking back and forth. A severely perforated bowel caused him so much pain that on a 1-to-10 scale, he rated it a 20. He was 87 years old and had been admitted 48 hours earlier with chest pain, but now the pain was localized in his abdomen. His daughter, Kathryn, had been called in during the night. Neither of them had slept.

Ray had to make a choice. If he chose surgery, it would have to be done immediately. Not having surgery would mean death. Ray's age and the magnitude of the surgery were two factors working against him. The surgeons couldn't guarantee a good outcome.

After Ray's pain was under better control, he lay stretched out on the bed, holding Kathryn's hand. They were deep in conversation, as if no one else in the world existed. There was no other family member to help them make this decision. I left them alone while I checked on my other patients; when I returned to Ray's room, he told me that he and Kathryn decided there would be no surgery.

He said it was an easy decision, and he was at peace with God. He'd lived a great life surrounded by the people he loved, and he had no regrets. If it was his time, it was his time. Kathryn appeared calm, strong, and remarkably comfortable with this decision. Whenever I asked if either of them needed anything, she always declined, saying, "No, I'm fine, thanks." Once I shooed her out to take a short walk to stretch her legs. She reluctantly went only after I promised to stay with Ray until she returned. I worried about her. I wasn't sure she understood what the next 24 hours would be like for her father.

The most valuable care I could give him was comfort. These would be his last hours on earth, and I wanted to make sure they were peaceful ones. I knew that as long as I kept his pain under control, Kathryn would be able to withstand the ending. After a few hours, Ray remained sleepy but alert. His condition worsened much faster than I'd anticipated, and although I was glad he wouldn't linger and suffer, I felt sad for the short time he and Kathryn had left.

When my 12-hour shift ended, I was asked to stay an additional four hours. Tired from such a busy day, I knew there was no one else to fill in.

Ray deteriorated quickly; his vital signs fell, and his extremities became cold and mottled. He didn't respond to voice or touch. His lung sounds were coarse and audible without a stethoscope. He showed no outward signs of pain.

It had been just Ray and Kathryn for years now. Ray's wife, Wilma, had died from cancer three years before. It was a long, harrowing illness. They'd been married 57 years. By evening I felt close to Ray and Kathryn, like they were becoming a part of my own family. I told Kathryn I would be her father's nurse until 11:30 PM. She seemed relieved.

Shortly after 11 PM, Ray took his final breaths and was gone. Kathryn was there, telling him it was all right to go. He didn't fight his death; he let it consume him peacefully. It was only then that Kathryn cried. We stood at his bedside hugging.

I left Kathryn alone with her father. It was important that she have the time with him to say good-bye. When she was ready to go, she thanked me for all that I had done for her father, even though I had played such a small part in this once-vital man's last days. When I got home that night, I was at peace with how that long day turned out. I, too, had no regrets. ▼

Florida Vacation

When a family can't bear to say goodbye.

Lorraine Randall, RNC

Marissa arrives at 4 PM in the oncology ward of my hospital. She can barely stand to walk from the wheelchair to bed. Her breathing is labored under her tremendous abdominal girth, and her hands and feet look painfully swollen. I apply a nasal cannula and she swats it away, mumbling. I glance at the orders; the admitting diagnosis scrawled on the order sheet: end-stage liver cancer with mets.

"We're here on vacation," her husband Anthony says. "My wife has been very sick. We just got married three months ago. We're from Staten Island, but her father thought the Florida sun might help her get better. We just got here and she's been real bad."

As I listen, I notice a "do not resuscitate" form attached to the chart. There's also an order for a morphine drip, which is needed immediately—she's agitated, moaning loudly, and struggling for breath. I explain to Anthony that we'll talk later after I make Marissa more comfortable and settle her into bed. Does he understand that she won't be going home, I wonder?

I find Anthony in the waiting room with the rest of Marissa's family. I whisper to him in the hallway. He holds his head so low that I strain to hear him. "The doctor says she's dying," he says.

I take his hand in mine. "It will probably be very soon."

"Yeah," he says.

"Does her family understand?"

"Well, they know she has cancer. But she didn't want them to worry. I'm not good at this. Can you talk to them?"

Anthony introduces me to Marissa's dad, stepmother, and younger sister. He returns to his wife's room, and I explain that Marissa has little time left. I suggest if anyone needs to be with her, they should come now. They gasp loudly, and I'm faced with incredulous expressions. Her father asks me, "Are you saying my little girl is going to die?"

I feel embarrassed at my reply. "I know this is a shock, but I believe time is of the essence. Do you need me to arrange for a clergyman?"

They all rush to Marissa's room.

I give them some time and then return to her room. Her family stares at me angrily when I enter. I'm accustomed to it—it goes with the territory.

And I'm okay with it because I hope someday they may appreciate my candor about Marissa's imminent death. Maybe they'll be thankful that they were able to spend those last moments with her before she died, instead of sitting in the waiting room hoping that she would get better.

Marissa continues to be incoherent, but her agitation has abated and her breathing is less labored. Her father follows me out of the room and asks me if I could be mistaken about her condition. "I don't think so," I tell him.

"Well, I'll talk to the doctor about that," he says. "Her mother is up in New York and won't be here until tomorrow. That will be plenty of time, right?"

I don't think so, but I tell him I don't know and that they should spend the night in her room or the family room.

When I arrive at seven the next morning, Marissa is in a coma. I find the family in her room as I make my rounds. Marissa's breathing is very shallow; she is close to death. I wonder how she made it through the night. Maybe, I think, she's waiting for Mom. Her family doesn't seem to understand she's in a coma and not sleeping.

When the doctor arrives they are waiting to hear him say that I have made a mistake, that Marissa is going to get better and leave the hospital. But the oncologist reiterates what I said yesterday. Softly but precisely, he tells the family he does not expect Marissa to hold on much longer. There is a collective sob from her family.

Within the hour Marissa's sister calls me into the room. "She's not breathing!"

I reach for my stethoscope, but before I can listen, Marissa gasps loudly. Her sister screams. Everyone else is silent.

Our hospital began a policy of playing "Twinkle, Twinkle, Little Star" over the loudspeaker with every birth. While I stand with my arms wrapped around Marissa's sobbing sister, the tune floats into the room as Marissa dies. It is 10:45 AM.

The family begs me not to move her until her mother can arrive. I place a DO NOT ENTER sign on Marissa's door and go about my duties. The day wears on and I am in the next room assisting in a central line placement. As I prepare to hand the doctor a syringe filled with heparin, I hear a tremendous wail. Hurrying next door, I find Marissa's mom draped over her daughter's body.

The family has arranged for Marissa to return home to New York City. It's 3:30 PM, less than 24 hours since Marissa and her family arrived at the unit. I offer my condolences and we embrace, and when they are gone, I accompany Marissa's body to the morgue. Getting off the elevator I hear "Twinkle, Twinkle, Little Star" from the loudspeaker again. ▼

In the Hand of Dad

Preemie's struggle becomes one nurse's journey with a father.

Sam Bastian, MS, APRN, BC

I suppose we are expected to welcome challenges in the neonatal ICU and, for the most part, we do, but when I heard that a 27-week preemie with multiple deformities was on the way, all I thought was, "Jeez, I could do without this." We were just reaching the hardest and longest stretch of the night shift when the call came-it was going on 4 AM-and because I had drawn the short straw, the next patient was to be mine. We immediately started preparing for the baby's arrival. Called respiratory to check the ventilator before connecting it to the bed. Got the pulse oximeter. Drew up meds. Got the warming lamps. Humidified the isolette. Got the stuff for footprints and identification bands. Pulled supplies. More information arrived: the mother was a pediatrician and the father a lawyer. I couldn't think of a worse combination of parents of a high-risk infant. The mom will know how things should progress, and the dad will be ready to sue if they don't go well.

Wallowing in self-pity and dread, I met the Flight for Life transport team. Their report: deformed limbs, difficult to ventilate, umbilical arterial catheter placed but not confirmed by X-ray, vitamin K in, silver nitrite in; pregnancy number seven for this couple, no living children, and the father was following in his car.

In the NICU, we began the dance of a well-rehearsed team. The neonatologist called out orders, and all available nurses ran blood, drew up IV fluids, entered information in the computer, and delivered X-rays. As admitting nurse, I stayed at the bedside, my hands in the isolette with the baby: *Push this, draw off that, take some photos for Mom, position for X-ray, adjust the monitors*. I hand-bagged intermittently as we tried to adjust the ventilator. The baby didn't seem to like any of the settings. When the respiratory therapist bagged, the baby's hemoglobin desaturated. I stepped in to bag again.

Dad arrived, Scrubbed and brought to the bedside, he stood on one side of the isolette. We exchanged introductions. The baby's name was Joshua, which means, "Jehovah saves." I filled Dad in on what little we knew. "We worry first about the lungs," I said. He nodded. "He's having trouble but we're helping him," I said. We both looked down at Joshua struggling to breathe. His entire body was barely bigger than my hand.

"None of our other babies made it this far," Dad said. "Some of them didn't even take a breath at all."

Joshua's oxygen levels kept dropping when he was placed on the ventilator. Hand-bagging was all that worked. After a while, the neonatologist told the respiratory therapist to relieve me. The pediatric pulmonologist driving to the hospital was at least an hour away. I stepped away from the isolette and the respiratory therapist took over, but when the oxygenation wouldn't stay within an acceptable range, I stepped back in and the level rose again. So there we were, Dad and I, standing two feet apart over his struggling son.

As he held Joshua's hand and stroked him, we talked about what he would like for his son. Joshua weighed only slightly more than a pound. Looking at him in the isolette, I couldn't possibly imagine him as a bouncing baby. His father spoke softly to Joshua: "Hang on buddy, stay with us awhile." After a few moments, I was really aware of only Joshua, his father, and myself in the room. Everyone was waiting for the specialist to arrive to examine Joshua and determine whether he would live. Other staff members asked me whether my hands were tired. Bagging continuously for 20 minutes can be uncomfortable, and I had already been doing it for more than an hour, but my hands weren't tired. Dad and I just continued to talk about how beautiful Joshua was. Yes, there were multiple deformities; his head was enlarged, his limbs twisted, his tiny hands had too many fingers, but we focused on the perfect parts: the delicate ears, the fingernails, and in between bagging, we caught glimpses of a sweet little face.

When my shift was over I didn't leave. I couldn't leave that baby clinging for life and the father clinging to his son. When the specialist arrived, I positioned Joshua for him and stepped out of the way.

Joshua died later that morning.

As I prepared to leave, exhausted and saddened, Dad excused himself from the bedside and called to me. "I want to kiss the hands that gave me time with my son," he said, bringing my hands to his lips. ▼

Inseparable

Bending the rules, preserving a vow.

Dawne De Voe Olbrych, MSN, RN, CNS

I met the Krauses on a Wednesday about 9 PM after Mr. Kraus had been admitted to the cardiac ICU. He was elderly and balding, and he had pale blue eyes that looked tired and frightened. "It's been a long night, huh?" I asked as I adjusted the O_2 tubing and snapped on the cardiac monitor leads.

He nodded, and then spoke in heavily accented English, "The pain in my chest was like a vise. It is better now. I am tired." He paused. "My wife? She is afraid. I can see her soon?"

"Absolutely," I replied, and assessed his vitals before going to look for Ms. Kraus in the waiting room. She was slender and petite, with reddish blond hair. She and I talked as we walked the short distance from the waiting room to her husband's room.

"My name is Dawne," I said. "I'm a registered nurse. After you leave, I'll take care of your husband until 11 PM, when the night staff comes on."

"I will stay here." She tightened her grip on the straps of her purse.

"You can stay while we get him settled," I said. "He has no pain now." I explained his status to her. "This monitor gives us a picture of his heart beating. A nurse watches it all the time. I've listened to his heart, and his blood pressure is normal. He has oxygen in his nose and an IV for fluid. Our visiting hours are from 1 PM until 8 PM, but you can stay for a bit as we get him settled."

It was my standard speech to reassure the patient and family, while acquainting them with the CCU and our rules.

We entered her husband's room and she immediately took his hand in both of hers and kissed his forehead. Their devotion to each another was visible. "I will stay here," she told him. He nodded and closed his eyes.

"You need to go home," I said. "Nurses are here around the clock. We'll watch his heart constantly. We will take good care of him. You need to rest. It's been a long night for you as well."

But Ms. Kraus was still by her husband's side when I left at 11:15. "You need some rest," I told her again.

"I stay here," she replied.

She'll get tired, I thought to myself. Maybe the night staff will be able to talk some sense into her.

I returned Friday after a day off and found Ms. Kraus sitting in the waiting room. She looked pale and drawn. "They are working on him," she said. "I wait until they are done."

I hurried into the unit, concerned that he had taken a turn for the worse. I asked the shift nurse, "Mr. Kraus?—"

"—is fine," she answered, finishing my sentence. "Small anterior wall MI, stable, ready for transfer out to the floor in the morning."

"His wife looks awful," I said.

"She won't leave," the shift nurse added. "She has been here since Wednesday night. Eats a bit off his tray, won't even go downstairs to the cafeteria. Sits in the waiting room when she's not in his room. I've talked to her till I am blue in the face, but she won't go home. She just sits there in that straight wooden chair and holds his hand."

I shook my head. How could she not go home? She needed to be well when her husband was released. We were pretty rigid about visiting hours; if something suddenly happened to him, she would be in the way. Families always ended up going home. She just didn't understand.

After report I found Ms. Kraus back at her husband's side.

"Ms. Kraus, your husband is doing well. The heart attack was small," I said. "He'll probably go home at the end of the week. You are exhausted." She shook her head but I pressed on, repeating what she had undoubtedly heard many times in the past 48 hours. "You have not showered, not slept, nor have you eaten properly since Wednesday. You'll be sick. You must go home to rest."

Ms. Kraus listened politely, and when I stopped for a breath, she put her hand on my arm and slowly pulled up her left sleeve.

"You can't—" I stopped midsentence when I saw a number tattooed on her arm.

"The only time we were apart was at Auschwitz," she explained. "I would not have lived if he had not been there on the other side of the compound. When we were liberated, we made a promise never to leave each other again." She pulled down her sleeve and took her husband's hand. "I have not left him since, and I will not leave him now."

At the nurses' station I told their story. The usual hubbub of the shift change abruptly stopped and quiet settled on the unit. Then we mobilized. Someone carried a basin and toiletries into the room so Ms. Kraus could freshen up. The secretary ordered a guest tray for supper. I draped a Barcalounger with a sheet, and found a pillow and a blanket. Thirty minutes later Ms. Kraus was asleep next to her husband's bed. Through the siderails their hands were still clasped.

Later during my rounds Mr. Kraus looked up as I took his vitals. "Thank you," he said quietly, "for finally listening." He glanced over at his sleeping wife. "We have quite a story, Stella and I." ▼

Steven

I still wonder if I failed you.

Karen Roush, MSN, RN, FNP

Your dying had started weeks earlier, but we refused to notice. It was late September. The shortness of breath, the protracted vomiting, the hours every morning emptying your bowels into the toilet before you could get on with the day. The emergence of bones everywhere, cheekbones and pointy shoulders and the orderly stacking of ribs.

You have been gone 15 years this week.

A phone call that morning sends me speeding to your house. I find you naked, wrapped in an afghan, confused, and lethargic. I help you dress and drive you to the hospital.

You are 26 years old.

That first night you slip into a coma, your thin limbs lying unnaturally straight beneath the sheet. The next morning I awaken in the chair next to your bed to find you sleeping, curled on your side, corticosteroids doing their magic on the swelling in your brain. Two nights later I'm running to the diner at 1 AM for burgers and fries, and now here we are eating popcorn and laughing.

You are more than my best friend. Have I told you that? I sit by your bed and wonder who I will laugh with, lament with, drink beer with on Saturday nights. Who will hug me, who will think me beautiful? I want to demand that this dying stop, scream at you not to leave. But instead I bring popcorn and videos and the Bazooka gum you love. And we laugh. Because even now, it is what we do best.

A nurse comes in, glares at us. "This is a hospital, you know!" and leaves, closing the door after her. We crack up. It becomes a running joke between us. We admonish each other repeatedly, "This is a hospital, you know!" "Oh, I thought it was the Four Seasons!"

It is mid-October, two weeks since your admission. After the first few days you have steadily worsened. We both accept you won't be going home again. Outside your window the sun shines on a glorious fall day. "Do you want to go outside?" You look surprised, not believing. "Do you think I could?" I want to cry with gratitude that there is something I can do after all, this small thing that has lit your eyes. "Sure, there's a porch off 2 East. We'll bundle you up in blankets." I find a wheelchair and extra blankets and soon we're rolling down the hall. People stare. I stare back, defying their curiosity, their fear, their health. Outside we sit silently, your face tilted to the sun, eyes closed. We stay like that until shadows envelop you and the air turns cold. "I'm ready to go back now."

You can't eat much anymore. Yet still the diarrhea is relentless. Sometimes it goes on for hours, I help you onto the commode, then back into bed, then a minute later, back onto the commode. It exhausts you. Soon you can't make it onto the commode in time. One night at 3 AM I help you into the shower, hold you up, wash away the accumulation of shit and sweat clinging to the remains of your body. You are 5′11″ and weigh 85 lbs.

You don't seem to fear death. You don't seem to fear the pain. But you are terrified that you will lose your mind. AIDS dementia, from the early days of your diagnosis you have dreaded that possibility. And now it has begun. You hallucinate, there are outbursts, disorientation. And then you will be absolutely clear again. It is during one of these lucid times that you ask me to kill you. You don't say it like that, you ask me to "help" you if things get too bad. "Don't let me end up like my grandfather," you say, having watched him die incontinent and demented. "I would do anything for you, you know that." I answer, horrified. "But you can't ask me to do that!" But it is too late, you have already asked.

You slip in and out of consciousness. Days and nights I sit, caress your shoulder, talk quietly into your ear. You're restless, moaning softly, one night you call out my name repeatedly. I had promised to take care of you. Now I sit by and do nothing while you lie diapered, delirious, suffering. I stare at the IV pump, watch the morphine drip. It would be so easy to accomplish what you had asked. ▼

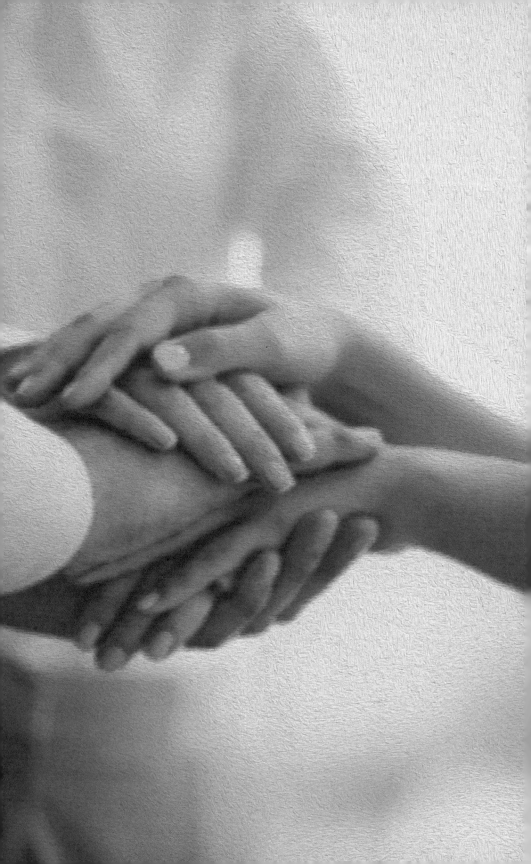

Colleagues, for Better or Worse

Stories of being helped or hindered, inspired or undermined
by colleagues. Learning better ways to
communicate with colleagues.

*"Each time, I remember the scorn of my
coworkers, and I feel a little jolt of
fear – just before I make the call I know
I have to make."*

Nancy L. Ball, RN

Roger's Angst

Why is it so hard for good nurses to move on from errors?

Evelyn Lawson-Jonsson, BSN, RN

He was standing in our small utility room—under the fluorescent lights, hands on the counter, head down. I started quietly backing out, thinking he wanted privacy. "Don't go," he said, in a low, gravelly voice. He shook his head slowly, as if in disbelief: "I have to give up nursing." Seconds ticked by as I wondered what could possibly be so serious. Did he have cancer? AIDS?

Roger was older than many on our floor, his coal black hair woven with gray. A quiet, competent leader with over 10 years' experience at our hospital, he'd served as a medic in the Gulf Wars. He was conscientious about his responsibility to his team members and patients, his performance reviews excellent. As the head nurse on the afternoon shift, he'd arrive early to organize his duties. His staff appreciated his calming influence during the sometimes frantic pace of our med–surg unit.

At last it came out: "I almost hung the wrong blood on my patient."

The words dropped like a curtain, leaving him with his thoughts, me with mine. I eased the door closed with my foot, already reviewing policies and procedures, looking for answers to the "how" and "why."

"But you didn't," I told him.

It sounded like a platitude, and Roger's response was full of self-loathing:

"But I could have!" Never looking up, he told me that he'd taken the lab slip to the blood bank, found the unit with the patient's name on it, but somehow grabbed the wrong one. He hadn't discovered his error until he'd checked the patient's name band.

"I could have *killed* my patient," Roger said, his voice thick with pent-up anger.

"Yes, but you caught your error," I said. "The blood administration protocol worked! There'd be no need for those last two checks if nurses were robots, but we aren't."

He didn't respond, so I pushed on. I told him that if he were the only medical professional to ever make an error, then yes, he should quit. But he had to be aware of errors others had made.

At this, he nodded slightly.

"You're an integral part of this unit," I said. "We need *you*; our patients need *your* expertise, *your* compassion." I fell silent. At last he looked up at me, through moist eyes, and nodded. My cue to leave.

After report, Roger came to me and requested the next day off as a "mental health day." I noticed that he had the following two days off as well, and hoped that during this time he'd regain some balance.

On the way to my car, I stopped in the cafeteria for a cup of tea. I found a table in a corner where I could decompress from the shift. However serious his error had almost been, Roger's conclusion to quit nursing seemed utterly irrational. And trying to help him gain perspective had left me drained.

Then an experience of mine came rushing back in full color. Early in my career I'd taken a position at a new hospital. I wanted to make a good impression. Instead, I made a serious medication error. I remember the terror I felt, the mixture of shame and fear as I filled out the incident report. Later that night I lay silently crying, feeling so ashamed I didn't even tell my husband, denying myself the comfort he would have gladly offered.

The next day, as I prepared my medication tray with shaking hands, two physicians sat at the nurses' station, talking too loudly as they discussed the medication error and wondered which nurse had made it. Overhearing them, I turned to confess, feeling like a marked woman. They muttered something in my direction, shook their heads, and quickly returned to their charting.

For weeks afterward I expected to be terminated. For years I told no one about my shameful experience. My "little secret" occasionally popped up, bringing a tightness to my chest, eating away at my confidence. Later, when teaching nursing students to pass medications, I didn't use my medication error as an example; my perfectionism wouldn't allow it.

As my tea grew tepid, I began to understand why Roger's response— and my own, for all those years—seemed out of proportion to the "crime." They were. Roger's expectation of personal perfection had blurred the mirror he used to evaluate himself as a nurse. What do conscientious nurses need when we make a mistake? Time to evaluate the situation, to learn from it—and then the healing salve of compassion from those who stand beside us, and those who lead us.

On the fourth day Roger returned. When he walked off the elevator, head held high, back straight, I felt certain his time off had been beneficial. He came over to see me at the nurses' desk. This time when our eyes met he said, with a sly smile and a sharp salute, "Roger, registered nurse, reporting for duty." ▼

The Blame Game

Judging patients for poor life choices is neither right nor professional.

Natosha Cramer, BSN, RN

I was just two hours into my evening shift as a certified nursing assistant when I noticed 12 missed calls on my phone. My mom, aunt, and grandma had been frantically trying to reach me, but my phone had been silenced. I called my mom right away. "Justin overdosed and is in the ICU at *your* hospital," she said as soon as she picked up the phone.

Justin is my cousin. A 28-year-old at the time, he had been in and out of jail since his teens, primarily for drug and theft charges. He had mental health problems, plus a congenital tremor disorder that had become apparent early in childhood. After age 18, he'd virtually vanished from the family. We knew that he was living with friends, but we otherwise had no contact with him.

Even though I hadn't seen Justin in nearly 10 years, my gut twisted at the thought of what condition he might be in. Was this overdose purposeful or accidental? I searched for answers that I knew I wasn't going to find. I had to go see him. My supervisor, seeing the sadness in my face, didn't ask any questions as she granted me an early dinner break.

I'd been to the ICU many times, but this time was different. I was no longer a hospital employee, but a patient's family member. The front desk secretary directed me to the room at the end of the hallway. Outside the room, I was approached by Justin's nurse, who introduced himself as Robert. I reciprocated the introduction while peering through Justin's window to see if I could catch a glimpse of him. It had been so long since I had last seen him that I wasn't sure if I would even recognize him.

The nurse explained that Justin had been found unconscious in a cemetery earlier that day. After receiving CPR and being intubated, he'd been transferred to the hospital, where it was determined that he had consumed a large quantity of alcohol and muscle relaxants. "Is he going to be okay?" I asked.

Robert shrugged. "Was he on any other drugs?" he asked.

I explained that there was a rumor that Justin was on drugs, but I wasn't sure.

"So you're telling me," said Robert, "as a member of his family, you're not sure what drugs he's on?"

I was stunned. What kind of question is that? I thought.

"I'm not very close to him," I told him.

"Well, this is what happens when you take drugs—you end up in the hospital hooked up to all sorts of monitors and a machine that's breathing for you. How stupid. Didn't he know that you can't mix those things together?"

I wanted to tell him how selfish and unprofessional he was for even mentioning such a thing when my cousin was just on the other side of the door, grasping at whatever was left of his life. Instead, I turned away, opened the door, and went into Justin's room. I was relieved that Robert didn't follow me. My gaze was drawn to the heart monitor on the wall, softly beeping at regular intervals. The room was cold, with a strong scent of bleach. Just as I'd imagined, Justin had multiple tubes coming out of his inert body. I sat, tears streaming down my face.

Soon my mom and aunt entered the room with Robert. I stood up to hug them. With uncertainty, my aunt asked, "What's going to happen next? Will he wake up?" I knew she was really asking if Justin was going to die.

"It's unclear what his prognosis is just yet," said Robert. "However, if he does get better, with cases like this they tend to go home, get back on drugs, and bounce right back into the hospital."

My mom, who is quite forward, responded that Justin wasn't perfect, but he deserved to be treated with respect. "If this is going to be a challenge for you," she said, "please let us know so we can request another nurse to work with us." After a long silence, Robert apologized and excused himself from the room.

My dinner break had come to an end and I had to return to work. The rest of that shift, all I could think about was how angry I was with Justin's nurse. How could a nurse be so heartless as to insult a patient in such a vulnerable state? There seems to be a dangerous epidemic of clinicians blaming patients for their health issues. As a nursing student, I saw more and more of this attitude. The health care profession seems to have evolved a culture of accusation and attack against patients, a group we should be empowering and protecting. One day, I hope to see a change in the way we view health and illness; otherwise, situations like the one I experienced will continue to occur. ▼

Who's the Fool?

No laughing matter.

Nancy L. Ball, RN

Jim had long, greasy hair, a scraggly beard, and long, yellow fingernails. He always greeted the nurses at the dialysis center with a warm hello. Whenever anyone asked him why he didn't cut his hair or beard, Jim replied that he had no money for such things. Since I cut my father's hair, I offered to do the same for Jim. I shaved his head and face and he seemed pleased to be rid of the hair. After that, I became his barber.

When Jim could no longer afford his private nursing home, he was moved to a larger, state-funded home. Several months later he was hospitalized for a stroke. Since the dialysis center was attached to the hospital, I performed dialysis on him as an inpatient. That day he was delirious, thrashing about on the bed, unable to recognize me.

After his hospitalization, Jim returned to the nursing home. From then on, he seemed more talkative during his visits to the dialysis center. One day I overheard his primary nurse say Jim had told her he'd been hearing cries from his nursing home roommate at night and could see one orderly holding him down while the other climbed on top of him.

When I cut Jim's hair again, he told me he was afraid to return to the nursing home. Each time he came he reported similar incidents. I began to wonder what they could be doing at night. Baths and dressing changes are usually done during the day.

It was 1993 and abuse of the elderly was just beginning to receive media attention. My sister has a friend who investigated claims of abuse in nursing homes and told us stories that made me take Jim's fears seriously. I asked to have Jim assigned as my primary patient so I could keep closer tabs on him.

Months passed, and Jim pleaded with me to do something. "I can see their shadows through the curtains," he said one day. "It looks like one is holding him down, while the other is on top. He screams and cries! Then the other day he just disappeared. I'm afraid they'll do the same thing to me."

I questioned Jim, trying to get names and dates that would provide me with evidence. The other nurses said Jim was just crazy, that he'd told them a similar story before. I wanted someone to back me up, so I spoke to his physician. He told me there was no evidence to suggest deterioration of Jim's cognitive ability since his stroke, but he offered no guidance as to what steps to take next.

I called the Elder Abuse Hotline and gave the representative all the information I had gathered. He gave me some guidelines for questioning the nursing home staff. I asked if he thought I was being paranoid, since Jim's mental state could be in question, but he told me they would rather investigate 10 invalid claims than have one missed incident result in suffering or death.

I called the nursing home director, gave her a synopsis of events, and asked her to look up the roommate Jim claimed to have heard being abused. I told her that the hotline staff would be following up on my complaint. She assured me she would investigate. When I told Jim what I'd been up to, he became more afraid than ever. I reassured him, telling him he would be safe, especially now that everyone was looking into the matter and watching out for him.

The nursing home director called to say that on the nights in question, Jim's roommate had been given a bath and evening care. The roommate had dementia and would frequently cry out at being disturbed. As for his disappearance, he'd been moved to another facility. A week later I heard from someone at the hotline that Jim's claims had been invalidated and the complaint dismissed.

The other nurses thought it was hilarious and chanted, "We told you so!" Even Jim's physician thought it was funny. Didn't I feel like a fool? he asked.

When I told Jim what I'd been told in response to his claims, he looked at me and said, "You know, the other night I looked out my window and saw someone dragging a big plastic bag across the yard. I think it was a body. I think they chopped someone up and put them in the bag to get rid of them!"

Since that time, I have reported other cases of elder abuse, all of which were substantiated. People now take suspicions of abuse more seriously than they did 15 years ago. Still, the sting of past embarrassment haunts me, stiffening my resolve to investigate every possible avenue before calling in a case. Each time, I remember the scorn of my coworkers, and I feel a little jolt of fear—just before I make the call I know I have to make. ▼

Ordinary Things

What gets you through the night shift?

Cindy McCoy, PhD, MSN, RN-BC

Carol's patient is in ventricular tachycardia again. In her 70s, the patient's been without brain function since she went into cardiac arrest while singing in her church choir. When I hear Carol call to me, I raise the side rail on my patient's bed, hurry across the cardiac ICU, and snatch the crash cart. As I shove it close to the bedside, Carol grabs the defibrillator paddles and shocks the patient. When the monitor shows no change in rhythm, Carol delivers another shock. This time it works; we watch for a minute to make sure the rhythm continues, then Carol goes to call the physician while I check the patient's IV, endotracheal tube, and urinary catheter.

We're understaffed, with six patients between us. Sometimes, at the start of a night shift, it's hard to feel positive when you know it might not be possible to provide the best care. We're several hours into the shift now, and saving this patient's life feels good. When Carol returns with her orders, we quickly prepare the medication and the new IV infusion.

I return to my patient, who has dozed off, then make a hasty round of the other patients: an IV bag needs to be replaced, a patient needs assistance onto a bedpan, another needs to be repositioned.

Since Carol's patient seems to have stabilized, I make a trip to the waiting room outside the unit. As I open the door several sets of sleepy eyes question me. I always dread this part of the job. No one wants me to call her or his name. I beckon the patient's daughter to the door, quietly explain the event, and ask her if she'd like to come in and talk to her mother. She smiles and follows me onto the unit. Even though her mother is sedated and on a ventilator, the daughter stands and talks to her, stroking her hair, holding her hand. I leave as Carol comes in to speak with the daughter.

My total-care ventilator patient needs a bath. I've cared for him every night for two weeks. In his early 60s, he crashed his car after a myocardial infarction. Since then he's had heart failure and acute respiratory distress syndrome and now has an abdominal dressing because of an infection at the site of an exploratory laparoscopy.

I can tell from his expression that he's depressed. Some of the other nurses don't like to work with him because he can be irritable if you do things for him without telling him first. I figured this out early and we get along fine. He's awake and alert and communicates well—mouthing words and using hand gestures—even with his tracheotomy tube. He likes to watch country music videos; we turn the TV on and I sing along. As I perform tracheotomy care and change his abdominal dressing, I talk to him about his family, their pets. After I bathe him, he and I decide that we will try sitting him up in the chair for a while. His wife usually comes in at about 6:30 AM, and we plan to surprise her. Carol and I enlist the help of the respiratory therapist, and together we help him up into the chair at the bedside. Although I have much to accomplish before the end of my shift, I decide to wash his hair and shave him. When he is clean, groomed, and smiling, we prop him up. He seems to tolerate it well.

The sun starts to come in through the windows. Carol makes a fresh pot of coffee. There's still a bag of dirty linens to empty, a drug cart to be exchanged, the schedule to review, and the crash cart to be restocked.

My patient's wife peeks around the unit's door at 6:30. Visiting hours don't begin until 9, but I always let her in early. I tell her we have a surprise for her. As she enters her husband's room, I watch from outside the door. His smile matches hers. I give them a few minutes, then go in. "Thank you so much," she says. She is crying. "He is going to be okay. I know it now. He looks like himself today."

I ask him if he'd like to go back to bed, but he says no. I leave them together holding hands.

Since I became a full-time teacher, it's moments like these that I miss the most—even more, maybe, than saving lives. ▼

Deception

Disappearing drugs and a fellow nurse in denial.

Corina DeVries, RN

"I've been fired," Janet sobbed into the phone. "Fired for stealing narcotics!"

I was outraged. Janet and I had been inseparable since nursing school. I knew her as a woman whose drug of choice was sugar and as a professional who regularly spent her break time comforting frightened patients. How could anyone believe she would take drugs intended to ease others' suffering?

"Janet is incapable of this," I told my boss, who knew both of us from nursing school. She agreed. Two weeks later Janet started a job at the long-term care facility where I'd recently begun working.

For the first month, our laughter rarely stopped. The absurdities of nursing—being spit on while giving medication, the funny things our residents said—became inspiration for hilarity. But our lighthearted camaraderie was soon dampened. One day, we decided to go out for lunch and I asked Janet to drive. I was shocked to find her new red sedan littered with empty soda cans, fast-food wrappers, and torn papers. Pushing some garbage aside to sit down, I uncovered an empty pill bottle of Tylenol 3. The name on the container wasn't hers. A strip of empty Percocet wrappers, still connected as if someone had removed all three doses at one time, lay nearby.

I was shocked. All I could do was hold up the empty strip and ask, "What's this?" Calmly, she replied that her brother had been hurt and an ED physician sent him home with Percocet because it was too late that night to go to a pharmacy. The Tylenol 3, she said, had fallen out of her daughter's diaper bag after a visit to her father's house. Wanting desperately to believe her, I let the subject drop. But the more I thought about it, the less I believed her. Two days later, I called her. "If you have a problem with drugs," I said, "I'll help you." She brushed off my concerns, repeating her explanations.

As weeks passed, I noticed Janet was liberal with narcotics, often dispensing them to patients with dementia and to those who hadn't taken them in more than three months. Narcotic consumption among residents increased substantially—at least on paper. I later found out that Janet's patients cried out in pain, yet when other nurses cared for them, they were unable to be roused for hours after receiving meds.

Even though Janet didn't seem impaired, I became increasingly troubled. Then an entire supply of Percocet disappeared from the contingency supply during her shift. Again, I confronted her, offering to help her get treatment. And again, she swore she was innocent, cooly reassuring me, "I would never steal drugs. I don't even get high off them like other people do."

Counts were often off by one or two pills during the weeks that followed. Although Janet was the only common thread in each of the discrepancies, there was no other evidence of her guilt. I was a coward. When offered an excuse to leave—a new job at a different facility—I took it. It was easier to leave and hope the situation would resolve without my input.

An air of suspicion settled over my old facility. Janet called often with details. Staff underwent drug testing and narcotics could be dispensed only when witnessed by two licensed nurses. Although Janet told me her drug tests had been negative, I heard from another friend that Janet's results were positive. The friend also related Janet's explanation: a prescription for Vicodin from previous ear surgery. In fact, I knew the surgery had occurred nearly six months before—could she still need that prescription?

Then Janet told me that an entire card containing 30 doses of Percocet had disappeared from the med cart of a 70-year-old nurse who'd been practicing for decades. Janet was the only other nurse on the floor that day. I could no longer deny her guilt. For the third time, I confronted her; for the third time, she denied everything. I hung up the phone and cried. Then I called Anne, Janet's supervisor, and told her what I knew.

Janet was fired a few days later. Anne called to tell me that an attempt to use video surveillance to catch Janet stealing narcotics had failed, and without evidence the facility was unable to terminate her for theft. They decided to fire her for divulging confidential information about the investigation—to me.

My heart sank. I should have shared my suspicions sooner. By trying to preserve our friendship, I had allowed my biases to determine my actions and share the blame for the suffering of our patients. And in the end, after all my efforts, my involvement was still the reason she was fired.

Since Janet's departure, the narcotic counts at the facility have been correct. Patients no longer cry out in agony. And I haven't heard from her. ▼

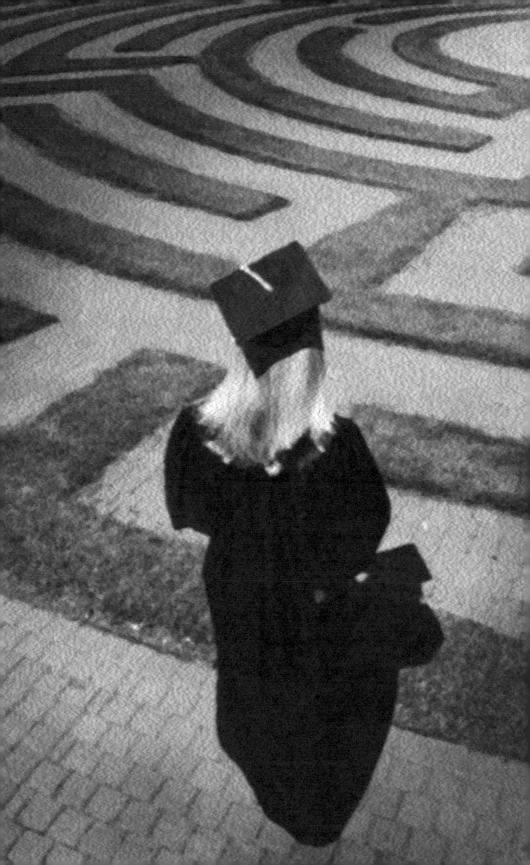

Career Is a Forking Path

The various dramas, status issues, and challenges faced by nurses moving into new specialties, leaving bedside nursing for management or to pursue an advanced degree before returning to the profession. And those returning to it after many years away.

"It wasn't easy to start over in a new job after all those years. But the rewards have been worth the risk."

Cortney Davis, MA, RN, ANP

The Fine Art of Leaving

The patients were the story—what was left was just a job.

Cortney Davis, MA, RN, ANP

S everal months ago, I handed in my letter of resignation at the women's health clinic where I'd worked for more than 16 years.

The letter said, in the words behind the words, that in a few weeks I would no longer drive each morning through the suburban streets, listening to *Morning Edition* on National Public Radio; no longer park my car in the basement of the gigantic hospital lot and walk up the cement stairs, stepping over cast-off Band-Aids and crushed-out cigarettes, following the signs that said, "Women's Health Center." I would no longer unlock my office door, greet my staff, and peer into the crowded, noisy waiting room. I would no longer know which of our patients would be blessed by successful pregnancies or negative Pap tests and who would be cursed by blighted ova, infections, or suspicious findings. It was easy enough writing the letter; it wasn't so easy leaving the job.

I've always found great joy in being a nurse. As a new graduate, I worked in intensive care, surrounded by monitors, ventilators, and central lines, the mechanical great grandmothers of the complex pumps and lines I see in the ICU today. Then I became head nurse on the oncology floor, the place where I learned when to bow to death, making way when he slipped in the door. Oncology, like the ICU, was a *body* place, a place of skin and blood, a world of intimacy and urgency where, if you weren't prepared to use your mind, your hands, and your heart, you wouldn't make it.

After several years, I returned to school to become an NP, which was still a new specialty. For the next decade I worked with pulmonologists and cardiologists in a subspecialty practice, then in family practice, and finally in 1991 I took a position in our local hospital's women's health center, an outpatient clinic for the uninsured and the undocumented.

Here too, I was working in a place where the body and the spirit were everywhere in evidence. Our patients were the poor, the women who could barely scrape together the rent and the girls who lived in cars or flitted from man to man to stay alive. They might speak English or Spanish or Farsi or Vietnamese; they might have only one pair of shoes or they might come in wearing spangles and heels. Whether my patients were abused women, abandoned mothers, or struggling addicts, I tried to accept them as they were. I especially remember Joanna, a young woman who confided that she had been abused as a child. Our ongoing clinical relationship helped her find counseling and physical and emotional healing. I believe that I helped my patients change their lives.

Then, about four years ago, other things began to change. There was increased pressure from insurance and managed care to cut costs and increase documentation, pressure that slowly filtered down to the clinical level in the form of budget reductions and cost-saving strategies. The expectation of upheaval was in the air. Which caregiver among us hasn't felt those strange vibrations?

If a floor nurse left a position or retired, that job was not always refilled. A few floor nurses, burned-out, resigned to pursue other careers. Expectations shifted, and every nurse had to do more work in less time. For a while, though, our little outpatient clinic seemed immune. We had a small staff and often seemed to fly below the radar.

Then the nurse midwife in our clinic was let go. We were all stunned. *How could this happen?* she asked me. The next day, my supervisor called me into her office. Our conversation went something like this:

"For years," Pat said, "you've been the go-to person in the clinic. I'd like to offer you the position of clinical coordinator. You're already doing most of the job."

I didn't answer right away. Why ask me to do what I already did? "That's okay," I said. "I like seeing patients. I like doing what I do now." Pat smiled. "We'll talk again," she said.

The following week, her smile was gone, her manner formal. The offer, she said, wasn't actually optional. Either I became the manager of the clinic or in three months she couldn't guarantee that I would have a job at all.

In my mind, I saw a silent parade: all the good nurses being marched away. All the nurses who really knew how to tend patients hustled from the bedside and yoked instead to paperwork and computer screens. All the experienced nurses, the ones who could recognize the stroke, the heart attack, the malfunctioning valve, the impending skin ulceration, the cyanosis, the swelling, the about-to-happen tragedy—all those nurses now overwhelmed, too busy, too focused on numbers and forms to minister to the patients. Was this my fate?

I took the position. Like other nurses, I needed the paycheck, the benefits, and most of all, the opportunity to serve. There were nods and handshakes all around. Then the weeks rolled into months and, little by little, my new job began to change.

I could no longer see patients. Budgets, scheduling, reviews, special projects, and hospital-wide initiatives filled my days. I put away my stethoscope, my white lab coat, my little notebook of facts and medication dosages. Patients and patient care receded until the concept of *caregiving* became only a pinpoint in the distance. Like other managers, I cut budgets and asked more and more of the already stressed nurses I had once worked alongside. Was this serving patients, supporting my staff, or upholding the words of my Nightingale pledge? Could I even call myself a *nurse?*

Then I noticed something else.

Writing has always been my avocation, what I love to do when I'm not working, and often my writing involves my nursing. But as my months in management became one year, then two, I realized I had stopped writing—during all that time, not one good poem and only rarely a finished story or short essay. The spiritual dryness I felt in my management role had invaded my writing life as well. Divorced from the immediacy of caregiving, I was cut off from the experience of *story*, from the human images and events that inspire me as a writer.

I handed in my resignation and soon began a new job in a new institution. This position offers less money and less flexibility, perhaps even less time to write. But I am, once more, where I want to be—with patients, doing what I've been trained to do, doing what I love.

I know no job is perfect; I will certainly miss the best parts of my time in the women's clinic. But I've learned some valuable lessons: I am, first and foremost, a nurse, in the old-fashioned sense of that word. I'm a tender of patients, face to face and skin to skin. In order to maintain this essential connection, I had to dispense with my clipboard and my portable phone, my calendar of budget meetings and deadlines.

I also learned that as nurses, we can sometimes become deadened to what we are doing. Whether we are staff nurses or clinical coordinators, we can become acclimated to stress, discomfort, compromise, and an ever-widening gap between us and our patients, one caused not only by insurance pressures but also by the steadily increasing demands of technology. Instead of taking care of patients, we manage their charts. Soon we begin to think that's what nursing is all about; we forget why we went into nursing in the first place.

It wasn't easy to start over in a new job after all those years. But the rewards have been worth the risks. Once again, I can pull up a chair and sit down next to the exam table. Once again, I can look my patient in the eye and ask, *how can I help you?* ▼

Making It Fit

A new NP on a psych unit finds her professional identity must be redefined.

Meredith Bailey, MSN, BSN, RN, PMH-NP

I work on an inpatient psychiatric unit and introduce myself as an advanced practice nurse or an NP. Often, patients look at me curiously and respond with something like, "So you're the head nurse?" Then I explain that no, I'm not the head nurse. I'm in charge of their treatment plan, medications, and discharge planning. This is followed by, "So you're like a doctor?"

Most of the time, I sigh and say yes, I suppose I'm kind of like a doctor. But my whole being rebels at defining my nursing practice as "like a doctor." I'm not a doctor. I'm a nurse. In my newest nursing role, it's been challenging to be trained by a psychiatrist and not initially welcomed by nursing colleagues. When I walked onto the unit my first day, expecting to be embraced by the nurses, I was dumbfounded and hurt that my own profession didn't accept me with open arms. The inpatient unit is a melting pot of professions, and I found that I didn't necessarily fit with the doctors, the social workers, or the staff nurses.

I was a new APRN, but I'd worked as a staff nurse in a pediatric ED for six years. I had been through a lot in the ED, personally and professionally. I'd come to consider my nurse colleagues as friends and teammates. We had each other's backs through the best and worst of times. In the chaos of an ED, it's imperative that the nurses unite, and we did. I'd assumed that this feeling of being a team carried across departments, hospitals, and roles.

I was wrong. There were staff meetings for nurses only and I wasn't invited. I was expected to go to medical staff meeting weekly—except on the weeks when the meetings were physicians only. I received a message, loud and clear, that I was something different, and I didn't like it.

I didn't experience nurses "eating their young." It was worse—they ignored me. At first I cried. I left each night feeling like I'd made a mistake in leaving the ED and entering this new role. I didn't want to be an APRN. I wanted to go back to being an RN. I felt like everything was backward. I now had residents and medical students following me around and doing rounds with me. My only experience with residents up to that point had been in the ED, and certainly not in a supervisory role.

It took time and a lot of patience, but eventually I started to accept and engage with my new role. The attending I work with is a psychiatrist and we often have nurse versus doctor debates. He helps me become an independent practitioner and I help him be more like a nurse. He also helps me navigate the challenges presented by my patients, the unit, and the hospital.

The medical consulting APRN also befriended me, and after my first month I told her my worry that the other nurses didn't accept me. She bluntly told me I wasn't a staff nurse anymore, so I should buck up and things would get better. That felt like nurse advice, and I didn't feel so alone any longer. Realizing that I couldn't be the only person experiencing this, I started to organize a meeting of all the psychiatric APRNs at the institution.

During my second month, some of the nurses realized that I could put medication and diet orders in and that I'm more accessible than my attending, so a few started speaking to me. During my third month, there was a seizure on the unit and I was the only provider on the floor. I handled myself well, and after that all the nurses began talking to me. I have done blood draws on hard sticks on the unit, and I drop by electroconvulsive therapy three times a week to place ivs so I can keep my skills up. It took time and energy, but I proved that I'm not scared to get my hands dirty and I'm definitely not "like a doctor."

After six months, a few of the nurses invited me to dinner. I immediately accepted, and while we were having our meal we talked about the difficulties they'd had with me and I'd had with them. We laughed because it seemed silly now, but in the beginning they didn't know where I fit into their world and I didn't know where they fit into mine. But I knew I was going to make them fit—because, like I said, in my heart and in my practice, I'm a nurse. ▼

Intensive Care

The author finds his ideal of nursing care in an inpatient hospice.

John B. Fiddler, MSN, RN, ACHPN

My first job as a nurse was offered to me by the director of a prestigious intensive care unit in the heart of New York City. He was enlightened enough to recruit novice nurses directly into critical care.

I spent the next seven years learning the ways of the ICU. I became expert at tending to the critically injured—and to the families who so often suffer alongside the patient.

I learned to balance potent resuscitative drips with human vital signs, bright red numbers and undulating colored waves upon a bedside monitor.

Family members would watch the waves, trying to make sense of the connection between the screen and their loved one lying in the bed beside us. Occasionally, the waves would decrease in frequency, then slow and fade into an unending flat line.

I experienced the power of critical care, of saving and extending life, and occasionally, prolonging dying.

I became comfortable with the power of silence, my presence as a nurse enough to reassure a family in distress. The simplistic-sounding components of therapeutic communication, learned in nursing school, became actively powerful.

"John, this is awful."

"Yes, Beth, this *is* awful."

I learned the truth will not kill you.

My interest in end-of-life care grew. I joined a palliative care committee and further explored the landscape of death and dying. I observed the ongoing legal and societal dyspnea provoked by a do-not-resuscitate order.

I have vivid memories of frail elderly hands—sometimes gently assisted—scratching a signature on a proxy form that could mean the difference between an uninvited intubation and the freedom to breathe (and cease to breathe) without mechanical assistance.

As a new NP, I was offered a position on a palliative care consult team. I knew I was edging closer to my ideals of nursing, of caring for patients and families in distress.

Challenges remained—I learned how to absorb instructions such as, "We want you to fix his pain, but don't talk to him about his prognosis."

A consult was canceled because the patient's presumed imminent death at the hands of a palliative care team would be reflected in a surgeon's mortality statistics. I witnessed relief from suffering withheld by medical staff and family members out of unfounded fears of opioid side effects.

Then, last year, I was offered a job in an inpatient hospice.

Inpatient hospice to me was the room at the end of the palliative care corridor that I had never bothered to visit. I had pictured it as a quiet haven for the dying, where birds chirp outside and music is heard playing through open windows as patients calmly drift off and up into dusty shafts of sunlight.

Not quite.

Instead, picture a unit where patients arrive on stretchers in extreme pain and distress, afraid, breathless—usually with families trailing behind, holding on to as much emotional and personal baggage as they can carry. Often these patients bear the physical and psychic bruises of a prolonged ICU stay.

And this is what happens here…

We do vital signs once a day. We examine *the patient* to get the information we need. There are no bedside monitors; the only waves we watch and negotiate are those of emotions. We address uncontrolled symptoms with a freedom derived from familiarity with the palliative effects of potent medications. We give antibiotics, place ivs, send labs, and will transfuse blood—but only if we think the interventions will help us ease pain and improve the quality of the patient's life.

Sometimes we do little, except remove the sticky layers of medications accumulated over months and years.

We see families liberated by a prognosis:

"Your mother has days to live… "

"I knew it, but no one ever spoke it. Thank you."

We see patients return home, renewed, able to complete their journey symptom-free. Others will die, peacefully, and we will scatter rose petals on their crisp sheets.

Our floors are carpeted and quiet. Indeed, we have a musician who plays guitar and sings requested songs at the bedside, and social workers and chaplains and volunteers who transform the clinical care into something wonderful.

And yes, I get involved in patients' lives, cry with them and for them, and yes, it is sad. But there is often a strong current of beauty and truth running within and alongside our dying patients that is missing in so many other areas of medical care.

For this intensive care nurse, nursing on an inpatient hospice unit is as close to the ideal of nursing as I have ever been.

And truly, I see now, the inpatient hospice is the ultimate *intensive care* unit. ▼

Am I a Nurse?

I'm old but never former.

Donna Diers, PhD, RN, FAAN

My RN licensure form surfaces in a pile of bills. For a moment, I wonder whether to keep my license active. It's an easy decision. Although I haven't touched a patient in a long time, it's still important to me to be licensed.

Since leaving clinical practice, I've been a faculty member in nursing and in public health, a dean of a school of nursing, and an editor of a national nursing journal—at times, all of these at once. But no matter my title, I've always been a nurse.

So what is my definition of nursing? Nursing is two things: the care of the sick (or the potentially sick) and the tending of the entire environment within which care happens. Throughout the years of changing job titles, the latter became my mission. The tending of the entire environment became more than an excuse for me to feel useful; it became the way I thought about the part of nursing that is central but invisible.

We nurses know how to get a patient discharged, how to get the right physician to show up, how to get the blood lab to pay attention, how to get a meal to a newly admitted patient in the middle of the night, where to find the secret cache of pillows, whom to call to get the defibrillator fixed, where the extra supplies are really hidden.

We know which surgeons to avoid scrubbing with, why the hospital is losing money on supplies, how patients are triaged from the ED to other units and counted in the census for billing, how mentally ill children wash through the health care system, why the work gets harder in the cardiac surgery intensive care unit when technology changes and stents replace coronary artery bypass grafts and the ICU fills up with "bellies" and trauma.

I currently work with a hospital finance department and decision-support team, mining the system's administrative data to contribute to decisions about practice, operations, and finance. The accountants and managers I work with are sweetly responsive when I can help them to see how their work might actually make a difference to the organization's patient care mission. I help them understand that the numbers they work with—the number of patients seen in the ED, enrolled in a special clinical program, or immunized for the flu—are not just numbers, but people. I've found that they want to better understand how things really work, even if occasionally my graphic description of the Whipple procedure stops the conversation cold and turns faces green.

Isn't this nursing?

It's clear to most of my colleagues that it is. I know that they see me as a nurse when they ask how they can make the health care system work for someone they care about. When a colleague is having trouble reconciling conflicting clinical feedback, I might be asked for advice.

I know that I'm a nurse when I mine the administrative data to help nurse managers or clinical nurse specialists make sense of and take credit for their work. I know it when I supply information that will help fend off a potentially stupid decision threatening to waste money and compromise the ability of nurses to deliver care. Through my work with data and data translation, I've become an advocate for patients and patient care.

So I'm moderately offended when one of my colleagues in finance refers to me as "a former nurse." I clarify: I'm old but never former. Still, I'm not on the nursing listservs for meetings and events or notices of deaths, wakes, marriages, and changes in positions. I'm not among those who are notified when something important happens. And (sob!), during Nurses Week, I don't get invited to the parties.

There's a whole underground of nurses out there, in business offices; in corporate compliance offices; and in decision support, legal, and informatics departments. For the most part, we don't know one another. Yet one of the joys of my present job is the opportunity to stumble onto these professionals. We recognize one another—nurse to nurse—by our understanding of how health care delivery really works. Most of us haven't left nursing, we've just broadened the definition.

There's no category on the licensure form for what I do, so I check "other." I'm an Other Nurse. ▼

A Moment of Grace

What is gained by the loss of a professional security blanket?

Cheryl Dellasega, PhD, CRNP

In 1976, shortly after our wedding, my husband and I relocated so that he could return to school. The ambivalence I felt about leaving my critical care unit job in the city turned to dismay when the tiny hospital in our new hometown informed me that they had no openings on their two-bed ICU, or any other floor.

In desperation, I interviewed at the Visiting Nurse Association (VNA) because I had agreed to be the breadwinner. The staff job they offered me felt like a demotion: I was an accomplished big-city critical care nurse with a superior knowledge of nursing, stuck with VNA nurses who didn't even wear white uniforms! Nonetheless, I grudgingly pulled out my high school sewing machine and made some uniforms out of the requisite blue pinstripe fabric.

My orientation was brief—for two days I made visits with others, then I was on my own. My new colleagues could charm their way past menacing dogs and cranky spouses; I was intimidated by the thought of drawing blood miles away from the nearest hospital, or figuring out if someone was in congestive heart failure without a monitor. I missed the electrocardiograph machines and ventilators that had been my professional security blanket.

One of my first solo assignments was to visit a woman named Grace. Grace was in her early 20s (like me) and had been diagnosed with schizophrenia; she needed Prolixin injections and nutritional counseling. Her chart was brief, noting only that she was noncompliant with oral medication and had a history of violent behavior.

She was considered to be an easy patient, although also a frustrating one, because nothing ever changed in her life, no matter what the VNA nurses attempted. My team leader considered Grace perfect for a "newbie" like me.

I thought otherwise. I had no experience in mental health, and, driving down the long, dusty lane toward her isolated home, I wondered if anyone would find my body buried in a haystack should something go wrong.

Grace turned out to be so rotund that she had trouble moving around the confines of her small world: a farmhouse where weeds exploded in the front yard and chickens scratched in the dirt out back. During our first conversation I gripped her slim chart and asked every question

I could imagine: "What do you like to do?" "How often do you go into town?" "What is your diet like?" "Do you have brothers and sisters?" Occasionally, Grace nodded a "yes" or shook her head "no," but mostly she just smiled. There were long stretches of silence.

After months of such visits, Grace began to talk—mostly about food. Sitting on the horsehair sofa in the parlor of the farmhouse, she would describe in detail the dinner she'd eaten the night before. Eating was perhaps her only pleasure, so encouraging a change in Grace's diet proved futile. In an effort to fill her time, I suggested a day program or a job. She smiled at the idea, exposing uneven, decayed teeth, but said nothing. I left a note for her parents offering to pursue the suggestion, but got no response. I never saw or spoke with them; they were always working on the farm. I seemed destined to offer her nothing more than a sympathetic ear.

The predictability of our visits became comforting to me. No matter how hectic my day, Grace's placid demeanor, her tiny voice, and the tick of her family's grandfather clock didn't change. I sensed she was happy to see me, too. When I arrived she was always waiting at the door. I began to understand that my willingness to be with Grace on her own terms was as healing to her as the IV medications I'd pumped into patients on critical care units. The insight that nursing was as much about relationships as about technical skills changed my professional focus completely. I decided that I wanted to get my degree and become a primary care nurse practitioner.

My last visit with Grace took place on a sticky day in August. Grace wore her usual faded housedress, Hush Puppy shoes, and gray ankle socks. When our hour together ended, she took my elbow and led me out into the humid afternoon.

A big truck overflowing with ripe watermelons was parked under a shady tree in the barnyard. The melons, from the farm, were headed to market. Grace chose one as firm and round as a basketball, brushed it free of dirt, and handed it to me.

We stood for a moment. Soon I would start classes for my bachelor of science in nursing and be reunited with old friends. Most likely Grace would remain in the remote farmhouse, spending her time eating or waiting for someone to visit. Our time together ended, as it began, with a long stretch of silence.

I climbed into my car, cradling the melon as I would a newborn infant. Clouds of dust followed my drive to the end of the lane. With one hand resting on the smooth, cool surface of her gift, I glanced in the rear view mirror, and saw Grace, standing by the truck, her hand raised in farewell. ▼

Promises to Keep

A 'routine' organ harvesting and a family's request.

Judy Morse, ASN, RN

"You have a harvesting for a patient in the ICU," said the voice on the other end of the line. It was Saturday, I was on call, and my morning routine—laundry, housecleaning—was officially over. This was to be my first organ procurement. I got in my car and began the 15-minute drive to the hospital. I had some idea about my role, but was unsure about specifics: What instruments would I need? Where would I get the ice? How long would it take? How would the family react?

Soon after arriving at the hospital, I began to prepare the operating room with Ruth. She and I had worked together since I began on the unit three years before. She was very experienced, which gave me some comfort, especially on call. I counted on Ruth to get me through.

As we gathered instruments and supplies, Elizabeth, the transplantation coordinator, came to brief us on the patient, a 45-year-old woman named Lynne who had brain death following a stroke. Her briefing was just that—brief—before she returned to the family.

When the transplantation team was ready, Elizabeth came to let us know. Ruth, the anesthesiologist, and I followed her to Lynne's room in the ICU. Family and friends surrounded her bed, visibly shaken, mourning the death that was to come. Some were crying, others were hugging, and one elderly woman sat quietly in the corner. I was unsure about what would happen next. Would the family leave before we wheeled Lynne to the operating room? Would they follow, as other families did? How could I walk over to the bed, unlock the wheels, and push the patient to the operating room as I had done so many times before? This time, there would be no return. I could not reassure Lynne's family that we would take excellent care of her.

Elizabeth introduced me to Lynne's sister. Instead of shaking her hand, I touched her arm. The three of us walked toward Lynne's bed, and Elizabeth told me of the family's request that Lynne not be left alone at any time. Her sister handed me a neatly folded pile of clothing—underwear; plain, dark slacks; and a long-sleeved, striped T-shirt—and asked that I dress Lynne after we were done. That's all they wanted.

Lynne's family stayed behind as we wheeled her out of the ICU.

In the operating room, I fell into my usual routine. Tending to the patient, keeping things in order, assisting the anesthesiologist, documenting—these were all tasks I had done many times before. As each procedure was completed the team grew smaller. Within two hours, Lynne's liver had been removed, the sutures were in place, life-support had been withdrawn, the medical team had gone, and Ruth had left to clean the instruments. I was suddenly alone with Lynne.

How little I knew of this woman. But there were tasks still to be done. I needed towels, warm water, and soap. I set out to retrieve them. At the door, I stopped and looked back. Lynne's body was exposed, alone in the big, empty room. I remembered her family's request. Returning to her bedside, I covered Lynne with a blanket, sat down on a stool beside her, and waited for Ruth.

Ruth returned about five minutes later. Noticing that the body and the room remained unchanged, she looked surprised. "I was waiting for you," I said. "We can't leave her alone." She smiled. Together we cleansed and dressed Lynne, then brought her to the morgue.

Outside the operating suite, Lynne's sister was standing in the hallway. She was alone. Without a word, she looked me in the eyes. I gave her a nod. She returned my nod, turned, and walked away. ▼

The Eyes of a Pediatric Nurse

Could lessons learned from children apply to adults?

Beverly Rossiter, MSN, CRNP, CPNP

Slowly, quietly, I entered 85-year-old Ronald Dixon's room. I was nervous. After 24 years as a pediatric nurse, I was seeing my first adult patient. As a professional, I knew the cries of a hurting baby, the stoic demeanor of the frightened school-age child, the need to put "Dolly" in a toddler's surgical bed as she headed to the operating room. But would I achieve the same understanding with my adult patients? Before starting this new job, I asked myself: Would what I knew about caring for children be of any use with adults?

As an admissions nurse, I didn't have to rush, and by habit I entered slowly and spoke softly. *Fast movement and speech can be frightening.* Mr. Dixon's reaction was my immediate reward—mirroring my relaxed demeanor, his dark eyes shone with warmth under a shock of bright white hair. Although frail in his white and blue hospital gown, his welcome was hearty. He introduced me to his daughter, Margaret, and his granddaughter Vicki. I shook hands all around.

Pulling a chair to the head of Mr. Dixon's bed, I sat down and looked into his eyes. *Standing over a patient can be authoritative or frightening.* He had chronic obstructive pulmonary disease and had been admitted from the ED with pneumonia. "I read the ED report," I told him. "It sure sounds like you've had some struggles. Why don't you tell me how you've been feeling?" As Mr. Dixon explained his medical condition, I touched his hand. *Show them you are not running away.* His speech slowed and his story gained clarity. He told me about his wife, who'd died only three years prior. They'd been married nearly 50 years. She had cancer, and he was her caretaker until the end. As he related the story he averted his eyes; I did the same. *Mirror the patient's tempo and temperament to establish rapport.*

I then turned my attention to Margaret and Vicki, who were standing at his bedside. Margaret was obviously troubled; she'd crossed her arms tightly and her hands were tugging on the elbows of her silk blouse. *Who else in the room is in need?* "It sounds like you've been having a rough time. You must have been really scared when his breathing trouble started."

Margaret described difficulties at work and problems with getting her dad to doctor's appointments. "His breathing's been bad, and it's getting worse. We don't know what to do anymore," she admitted. "You're doing the right thing," I reassured her. "Is there anything special that we should know to ensure your dad gets the best care?" *Family can provide invaluable insight into the patient.* We discussed his tendency to get out of bed at night without using his cane. She was comforted when she found that the bed alarm would ring if he was to make any major movements during the night. *Gain the patient's trust by gaining that of his caregivers.*

Finally, I performed assessments, explaining each step along the way. *Engage patients in their own care.* As I showed him how to use the pulse oximeter, I explained, "This helps us see how well you are breathing." Margaret interjected that his breathing trouble arose mainly at night ("We're always so worried when he goes to bed," she said). I assured her that we would watch his breathing through his monitor. *Remind them that comfort is always nearby.* My time with Mr. Dixon showed me that my pediatric eyes—trained to see what my young patients couldn't, or wouldn't, tell me—would remain invaluable in this new field.

Before I left, Mr. Dixon told a few jokes. His daughter had heard them a hundred times before—she rolled her eyes as he spoke. But at each punch line, we all laughed and laughed, like it was the first time. ▼

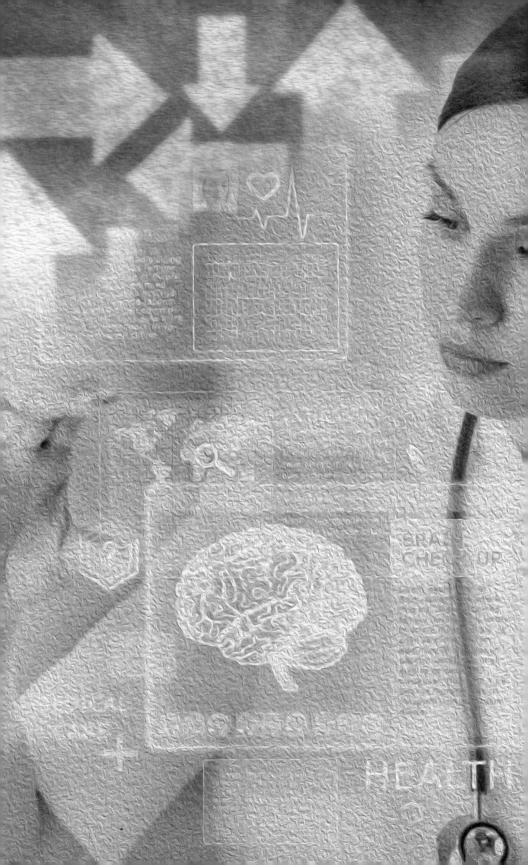

Connecting/Disconnecting

The conflicts arising for nurses adapting to new technology such as handheld devices, electronic health records, or bedside monitoring devices that can undermine direct experience with the patient. What makes us more or less human in all this?

"If you ask me today about cell phones, I will tell you a story about the power of a final connection, a eulogy echoing through space in hopes of finding one woman's soul."

Cynthia Stock, MSN, RN, CCRN

Before the Signal Fades

Patient and family cell phone use can seem intrusive in a hospital—until it's not.

Robbie Ravert, RN, RNC-OB

O
h no, here comes another dad with a Bluetooth.
      My colleague and I roll our eyes at each other in frustration. *Another self-important junior executive who must be in touch with everyone in the world while his wife labors unsupported*, I mutter with dismay as I rise from my chair to greet our newest birthing couple.

I have to coach myself: *Change your attitude. Change your attitude*, as I weigh the mom and escort the couple to the birthing room. Dad-to-Be proceeds to spread out his equipment on the dresser in front of the window while Mom-to-Be, in obvious distress, changes into a gown in the bathroom.

It occurs to me that I'm getting too old for this, as D-to-B struts about the room, speaking into the air. I spend the remainder of the shift trying to find ways to engage him in the care and support of his wife. I'm only partly successful: I teach him to apply counterpressure for his wife's back pain, but even in this he works with one hand, keeping the other on his computer keyboard.

While strolling in the hallway pushing her IV pole or digging in the freezer for an ice pop, he speaks loudly into the air, gesturing to an unseen business associate. I draw the water for her whirlpool. *If he only knew what he's missing. ...*

Communication technology has changed the culture of our birthing rooms in many ways. Consider the group of teenagers in the hallway, each one on a cell phone while their girlfriend labors; the new aunt with her feet firmly planted at the side of the infant care center while taking a picture with her cell phone; or the patient texting during a pelvic exam, while she miscarries. Consider the challenge of reviewing discharge instructions while all eyes go to the cell phone vibrating on the over-the-bed table, the educational opportunity vanishing.

By the end of the shift with D-to-B and his equipment, I'm thinking maybe we need to put up a new sign about cell phone etiquette. I'm even thinking we should ban cell phone usage altogether.

But one evening the patient is a young woman who's already been through three miscarriages and a stillbirth. Now, at 18-weeks gestation, she's bleeding and contracting. Her husband, a truck driver, is in the next state, at least three hours away. Her mother is frantically trying to contact him on the cell phone, while at the same time attempting to comfort her sobbing daughter.

Finally, the husband is reached. I'm told he's turned his truck around and is heading for the hospital. Labor is progressing rapidly, as I finish injecting a second dose of Nubain. The patient's mother is on the phone—as she has been almost continuously since she arrived. The patient begins to feel pressure. Her mother doesn't hang up, but she has to put the phone down momentarily so she can stroke her daughter's forehead and arm. One mild push and the tiny baby is in my hand, her heart beating visibly inside her tiny chest.

"She's alive!" her grandmother says.

I place the child's limp body on a towel and gently lay her on her mother's abdomen. In a second, the grand-mother is back on the phone; I watch in tearful disbelief as she puts the phone next to the baby's head.

I can hear the child's father repeating, "I love you, Daddy loves you," to his newborn child, from somewhere along Interstate 81.

I'd be lying if I said the sight of a Bluetooth doesn't start the growling in my head, or the chatter of several cell phone conversations outside a birthing room doesn't make me want to shut the door. But despite the irritations of communication technology, I have to say I'm thankful for the meaningful connections it sometimes does make possible. ▼

Paper Chart Nurse

Electronic medical records prove a stubborn technical challenge for a seasoned clinician.

Joyce Hislop, RN, OCN

In our oncology practice I am, at 68, the symbolic "golden girl" of a four-generation RN staff of six. My colleagues range in age from 25 to 50. Our lives and career experiences vary, but we share a passion for the challenges and advances in oncology nursing.

Always in my mind, however, is the uneasy, nagging sense that to these younger nurses I'm an old dog learning new tricks.

I joined the practice two years ago. During my initial interview, the office manager and the clinical coordinator were pleased with my oncology experience, but hesitant about my inexperience using an electronic medical record (EMR) system. Would I be able to achieve the proficiency level required? After spending time observing a nurse using the system, I told them I could learn to manage it.

Goodbye paper charts! Now I was the conductor of a desktop computer *and* a laptop—at first unable to quickly switch between the two EMR programs using a single computer, I needed two computers—plus a pager from the infusion room nurses that went off at annoying times and never carried any good news.

Several required computer orientation classes later, I was still entering and extracting information at turtle speed, the by-now-tattered EMR reference manual always within reach, my peripheral vision furtively searching out any colleague to ambush with yet another question. Soon I began cornering the market on Tums. Despite support and patience from management and colleagues, I felt my confidence and job security going down the tubes.

Staffing issues dictated that my orientation time be accelerated, and before the normal three months were up I was assigned to partner with a physician. Now I couldn't afford to dillydally over the keyboard. So I'd complete the patient care documentation portion of the EMR, but skip the billable service fields, thinking I'd fill them in later. Unfortunately, "later" became haphazard and then hardly ever. The billing department sent me daily agitated reminders to clean up the shocking number of data omissions and errors.

Near defeat, I initiated a conference with the clinical coordinator. She enlisted the help of a young systems operator. Tom (not his real name) came to spend some time with me at my computer. In retrospect, I see that he did the best he could with the raw material he had to work with. He was very good, directing his fingers unerringly over the keyboard as I struggled to observe each pathway he used and to jot it down step-by-step in my little black book. Flushed with embarrassment, I'd ask Tom to verbally walk me through something he'd just demonstrated.

After an hour he began to realize that I was still in EMR limbo. His attitude became a tad condescending, his directions bordering on sarcastic. I told myself he was a nice guy; he was just reacting out of frustration with his pupil. Gathering what little dignity remained, I stayed mute and coolly looked him straight in the eye. "Well, Thomas," I was thinking, "someday *you'll* be 66."

The electronic charting system became anathema to this paper chart nurse—at some point every day I'd want to either throw up or cry. After months of this struggle and continual dependence on coworkers to bail me out, I wrote a letter of resignation.

The manager and clinical coordinator considered my reasons and spoke to the other nurses, all of whom seemed to value my nursing experience over my EMR difficulties. Their suggestion was that instead of partnering with a physician, I do all the daily nurse visits, until now shared among the six nurses—a change that freed them up to focus on uninterrupted work with their assigned physicians. My role involves vascular access device lab draws and flushes, symptom management, teaching self-injection, and other nursing responsibilities. The EMR system for these duties is quite manageable. My dignity was spared, my confidence renewed.

I see many patients on a regular basis, and have developed their trust. If I'm not in the office on one of their visits, they'll mention it when they see me next. I still have the occasional mental block when completing an EMR entry or remembering an information source. Thankfully, my peers are never too busy to recharge my spirits. But I have to say, if this hospital switches to a different EMR system, it may be time to quit while I'm ahead. ▼

Final Connection

A nurse finds she must revise her negative view of cell phones.

Cynthia Stock, MSN, RN, CCRN

On Monday, if you had asked me how I feel about cell phones, I would have come up with this: I hate to listen to the drone of conversation coming from the person next to me on the treadmill at the gym. I don't care about trouble with the HOA. I don't care about a son who can't decide on a career as a director or an actor. I work out to smooth the kinks in my soul from a job that requires me to navigate a relationship with life and death.

Today, ask me how I feel about cell phones.

Yesterday my patient died. It was not an easy death for her. It was even harder for the family. The woman's adult children researched and found interventions not available in a small town. They urged their mother to seek treatment, even though it meant leaving home and the things that made her special. You know the things: a workroom filled with boxes of fabric, a classic cookie press, an old Singer sewing machine still made of metal parts.

For love of her children she traveled several hours and agreed to a procedure full of risks and potential benefits. Everything that could go wrong did.

After several days of watching their mother deteriorate, the children needed to go home and attend to their own health and home maintenance responsibilities. The day before their mother died I suggested they wait until a stable 24 hours passed. She had been improving, but she remained unresponsive, except for a rare flutter of her eyelids. I labeled her physical condition tenuous.

I started my next shift at 7 AM. In less than 10 minutes, I knew I needed to call them back to the hospital. I dialed the daughter's cell phone and found that she and her brother had gone all the way home, not to the motel where they, like their mother, had been suffering their own sort of displacement.

I knew their mother would die sometime that day. The thought of such a loss, handled long distance, tormented me. Haunted by images of my mother's last foray into the hospital, I recalled my fear of her suffering some catastrophe with neither me nor my sisters present.

Several phone calls took place between me and her children, her children and her physicians. While we talked and planned, rationalized and apologized, the patient's kidneys failed. She stopped responding when I called her name. The most extreme efforts to maintain life began to falter. The children's only request was to say goodbye to her.

This time I called upon the cell phone, the villain in a world filled with too much information and not enough direct human contact. I set a time for the children to speak to their mother.

I have big hands. A cell phone feels so small and thin. I have to concentrate to dial. I invested in a TracFone for 911 calls or lesser emergencies on lightly traveled roads, not for heavy conversation. For that I stick to my landline. So my supervisor's phone facilitated the last goodbye.

I called the children and put the phone on speaker. "I'm holding the phone to your mother's ear." Picture a frail octogenarian, skin gray, loose, with patchy bruising along her forearms. She seems asleep due to a continuous infusion of sedative. Tubes, tape, and devices defile the facial features that make her someone's mother.

The daughter's words stuttered from a bad connection, conveying a simple, beautiful tribute to a woman who created art just by being the mother to two children.

"Thank you for being such a wonderful mother. Thank you for being there and teaching us how to be good people. Thank you for loving us so. I know you have just moved on and will be waiting for us in a place where we will all be together. I love you, Mom."

I heard words I might someday say to my mother. I sucked in a breath but couldn't hold back my tears. I hoped the children didn't hear them.

"Here's brother."

From the phone came the sounds of the phone being passed. A male voice, sobbing, announced, "I love you, Mom."

What passed between mother and children through a lightweight assembly of black plastic pieces felt no less painful or final than if they had been standing at the bedside. I felt the privilege of having shared such a moment with a unique family. I cried as if they were in the room, quietly, so as not to diminish their pain with my own.

If you ask me today about cell phones, I will tell you a story about the power of a final connection, a eulogy echoing through space in hopes of finding one woman's soul. ▼

Chaos

Seven patients, one half hour. They call this nursing?

Lorraine Dale, RN

Rounds begin with a quick check of my patients to see that they're all breathing and that nobody's in acute distress.

Patient number one, who has an admitting diagnosis of unstable angina, complains of chest pain. He rates it a 3 on a scale of 1 to 10. I put on O_2, call for STAT electrocardiogram (ECG), and give him a nitro. Vitals are good, color is okay, no diaphoresis. I make a mental note to check back in five minutes to see if he needs another nitro. I wish I could stay but I have to see other patients on the floor.

Patient number two, Mr. Van Zandt, seems to have been here forever. He has a tube in every natural and surgically created orifice. He's completely helpless. I have to reposition him because he's tangled up in the bed sheets, which hampers his breathing and puts him in danger of aspirating his tube feeding. I do the best I can alone, but he weighs 230 lbs. and is lying in his own feces. I'll have to finish these rounds quickly and then find someone to help me clean him. Patient number one still has chest pain, although it has abated, so I check his vitals and give him another nitro. The ECG still hasn't been done.

I go on to patient number three, Ms. Caldie, who was treated for pneumonia but is ready to go home. This should be a quick check, but as I walk in the door I see her sitting up, dressed, arms across her chest, with an impatient look. "I've been ready to go for half an hour," she says. A doctor discharged her while I was getting report. Now I have to do the paperwork and give instructions. I calm her a bit and convince her to wait another half hour while I finish my rounds.

Patient number four is still in the cath lab. I don't have to worry about him yet. Patient number five returned to the floor a half hour ago after having a cardiac catheterization. I check his groin for bleeding and hematoma. Pulses okay. Vitals good. I'll have to check his cath site every 15 minutes to make sure he's not bleeding. He needs to lie flat and still for two more hours but he's fidgety from pain, so I promise him medication before leaving his room.

I recheck patient number one. His chest pain is worse, his color ashen. I check his vitals and give him another nitro. His oxygen saturation is down, so I turn up his O_2. I finally get his ECG, which does indeed show signs of cardiac ischemia. I page the physician, anticipate his orders, and prepare to administer morphine and start a nitro drip. I finally receive orders to transfer him to a nearby hospital for angioplasty or bypass. I administer the morphine and the nitro drip.

As I move on to the next patient, I walk by Ms. Caldie, who gives me a dirty look.

Patient number six has Alzheimer's disease and has been admitted because of a gastrointestinal bleed. His hemoglobin is down to 8; he's getting a blood transfusion and a bowel prep before tomorrow's colonoscopy and cautery. I quickly auscultate his lungs and hear signs of congestive heart failure. I'll have to call the physician for diuretics. His hands are restrained because he keeps pulling out his IV; this one will need very close watching all night. My beeper goes off: the ED wants to admit a patient to Ms. Caldie's bed. I say I can't take that patient yet. I'll probably hear from the supervisor about this.

One more patient to check, but first I check patient number one again. Then I medicate patient number five and check his groin for bleeding. I walk past Mr. Van Zandt's room and notice his oxygen mask has slipped off. I feel bad knowing that he's still lying in feces. As I fix his mask, I consider giving Ms. Caldie her discharge instructions, but I better at least look at patient number seven first. I'm glad that I do because I find her halfway out of the bed, insisting on going to the bathroom. She had suffered a stroke the day before and hasn't accepted that she can't walk. She's oblivious to her IV, which has been pulled out in her struggle to get to the bathroom. I turn off the IV that's dripping on the floor and stop the bleeding from her arm. My pager goes off as I help her to bed: Patient number four is returning from the cath lab.

All of this in the first half hour of my day. Would it be too much to ask for better staffing and working conditions? It seems the administration can throw any working situation at us and just say: "Sorry, we don't have any more help. Just do the best you can." And I do. We all do. But I wonder if these seven patients would believe us. ▼

Heads and Beds

What's the cost of an hour?

Marie E. Lasater, MSN, RN, CCRN, CNRN

I have six patients this morning. One with a self-inflicted gunshot wound to the head who's expected to die on my shift. Two with recent strokes, one with a lumbar drain after back surgery, and one with a possible prion disease. The newest one, transferred last night from the ICU, recently had brain surgery. Because of a sick call, we have only one patient care technician for 20 patients. I will be doing total patient care.

I assess my sickest patient first—the one who shot himself in his home, in front of his family. They want to be called when he has died. His face is horribly disfigured from the gunshot. Although he's unconscious, I tell him my name and that he is not alone. I touch his hand and tell him that I will be with him for the next 12 hours. I remind myself to check on him as frequently as possible. I don't want him to die alone.

The brain surgery patient looks uncomfortable; I reposition him and elevate his head to decrease swelling. I assess his level of consciousness, strength, vision, and pupil size. In neurology, the smallest delay in treatment can result in brain damage. I crush his pain medication, put it in applesauce, and carefully feed him while watching for any signs of aspiration. I will come back and check on him to make sure it's working, and to reassess his neurologic status.

I next check on my patient with the lumbar drain. The tube must be manually adjusted to allow 5 to 10 mL of cerebrospinal fluid to drain per hour. I see we're behind schedule, so I adjust it. It's important to keep the spine in alignment after back surgery; I help her to turn by logrolling. I check her strength, pulses, sensation, and skin integrity. I will reassess the drain within the hour.

One of my stroke patients has a feeding tube, and her swallowing mechanism is impaired. She's also in isolation for a drug-resistant organism. I don protective gear, begin her tube feeding, and evaluate her using a stroke scale, which indicates that she's improving from previous assessments. Her stroke causes her to be impulsive, so I caution her not to attempt to get out of bed without help and I make sure the call light is within reach.

I get a page that I'm getting an admission, a soldier with a seizure disorder who's been sent here from the military hospital for evaluation. I will wait to see my stable stroke patient but I do need to check on my patient with altered mental status possibly caused by a prion disease. He is unable to communicate and is incontinent. I can smell that he needs help. I cleanse him and change his linens. I then go to admit my new patient.

I now have seven patients. According to our staffing grid, I should only have five patients. We jokingly call it the "heads and beds system," because how sick the patients are isn't taken into account. We're not allowed to staff according to potential admissions, only for those patients who are already on the unit. We've recently been told that the hospital has below-expected revenues, but the chief executive officer made over a million dollars last year.

My new admission is a young soldier who's been taken off the front lines for evaluation and treatment of his seizures. He tells me, "I just want to get back to Iraq with my buddies." Before I begin to assess him, I pad his side rails in case he seizes.

And he does. I carefully note that the seizure lasts 45 seconds, his right arm and leg jerk, he's not incontinent, his oxygen saturation and vital signs remain intact, and he can't speak for five minutes. As I'm paging the physician, I get a page that my stroke patient on isolation is getting out of bed. I get a page a moment later that the oxygen saturation level of my dying patient is dropping.

I race to don protective gear and help my stroke patient to the bedside commode and back to bed. I then check on my dying patient. I hold his hand for a moment. As I'm telling him he is in a safe place, that his family is safe, and that people care about him, I'm paged again: I'm getting another admission.

I have been at work for one hour and 15 minutes, but I haven't even begun to give scheduled medications. We were recently told that we will be "counseled" if we clock out late from our shifts. I tell the unit secretary I will be in my dying patient's room and ask the other nurses to handle my pages. I hold my patient's hand and keep repeating, "I'm here." ▼

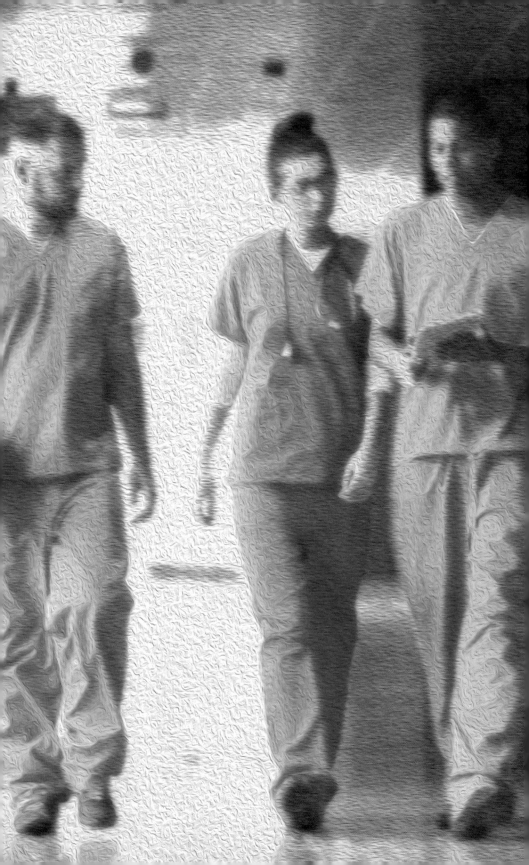

Lessons Learned

Stories about a nurse or a patient who is forced to reconsider assumptions about other people, the best approach to care, or their own perceptions or abilities.

"I saw then how easy it is to flatten our patients – to compress their personality into the framework of their needs. Those needs are never the whole story."

Meg Sniderman, RN

The Ice-Bag Incident

Was a loss made worse by nurses?

Kathleen L. Sitzman, MS, RN

On October 8, 2003, my dad had a massive heart attack at home. My mother called the paramedics, who did everything they could to save him, but he was pronounced dead upon arrival at the ED. Twenty minutes later, when I got to the ED with my mother, husband, and 15-year-old son, a social worker (who is a colleague of my mother's) told us the news. He also introduced my mother and me to the staff as "a social worker and a nurse" and announced, with a nod toward the ED staff, "These are the nurses who will be taking care of you today." The nurse assigned to us looked at me, then turned and walked away.

When we went to see my dad's body, there was vomit on his gown and tubes hanging from his mouth. Cremation had been planned, so I set about the task of cleaning him up. Two nurses stood in the doorway, watching silently. They left the room as I struggled to find supplies. When my mother asked for a lock of my dad's hair, I asked a group of nurses for a pair of scissors. They were perusing a scrubs catalog. One said she would find a pair "somewhere" and then went back to flipping through the catalog. Eventually a different nurse entered, handed me the scissors, and left the room, muttering instructions for me to leave them at the desk when I was done.

Just as my 12- and 17-year-old daughters arrived to say good-bye to their grandfather, the doors on the opposite side of the room flew open and a nurse appeared holding two Ziploc bags full of ice. I asked if the ice could wait for five or 10 minutes. "There are time limits on organ donor eyes," she replied, "and I must put the ice on now!" She placed the bags of ice over my dad's eyes, holding them in place by leaning on my dad's face with her lower arm and elbow, and then roughly secured them with an Ace bandage. When she was done, his hair stuck out in all directions. His right upper lip had been pulled up into the bandage, making it look like he was snarling. The bags weren't fully closed and ice water trickled down his chin and onto his chest and gown. I closed the bags, but not before his gown was soaked. I was too stunned and numb to fix anything else. This was my children's last vision of their grandpa.

A few months later, I contacted the hospital administrators and arranged to speak to the ED personnel during a staff meeting, hoping that by discussing my observations I might clarify for them what a family needs when a loved one dies.

When the ED director introduced me, postures stiffened and all movement came to an abrupt halt. With so many hostile faces turned my way, I paused, wondering if I had the courage to continue. I thought of my dad, my family, and my belief that every nurse sitting in that room wanted to do the right thing. I forged ahead.

As I described the ice-bag incident, a nurse sitting in the front row grimaced, her eyes wide. A nurse who was standing rolled her eyes and whispered to those near her. When another nurse said she would try to be more attentive to the families of dead patients, mumbling rippled through the meeting.

Although I made it a point to express my respect for their work, I heard many discouraging remarks at that meeting. One nurse commented, "Since you are a nursing professor, you probably don't know that ED nurses have no time for this kind of thing." Another said, "You obviously don't understand how hard it is for ED nurses to comfort the families of patients who have been dropped on our doorstep already dead." Still another said, "I don't understand what more could have been done for you. Did you need hugs or what? Warm, fuzzy behavior is not my style!"

My response to these nurses was this: "Hugging was not the point. I wanted the nurses in this department to pay attention to my family and me. I wanted the nurses to verbally acknowledge our grief. I wanted eye contact. I wanted help caring for my father's body. I wanted sensitivity when my children came to say their last good-byes. And I wanted basic respect and loyalty from my nurse colleagues. I do not think this is too much to ask."

When I was finished, the ED director thanked me for coming. Then he turned to the audience and said, "I know we all do a great job. Remember that this is just one family member who had a problem."

About three weeks later, I received a card in the mail. It was from one of the ED nurses, and it read: "Your willingness to help us, and teach us, despite the personal cost of reliving that experience, is most appreciated. Many nurses have approached me in the last few days, all resolving to change their nursing practice." ▼

Nurse, Heal Thyself

Walking in the patient's shoes.

Maureen Anthony, MSN, RN, CS, CDE

Ibecame a patient not by fate or genetics, but by choice. As a diabetes educator, I'm frequently asked to counsel patients having difficulty with the changes in lifestyle necessary to achieve blood glucose control. All too often the referring physician or nurse warns that the patient is "noncompliant." I've pondered the meaning of that word for the past three decades.

In my younger days, I thought noncompliant patients purposely ignored good advice while they blithely pursued lives of self-indulgence. Yet soon after starting work as a diabetes educator, I began to recognize the difficulty in changing lifestyles, even without the burden of insulin, glucose monitoring, and foot care. This understanding grew as I faced—and failed—my own comparatively minor challenges, such as how three pregnancies in less than four years left me with a few extra pounds to lose. I vowed "every day" to start "tomorrow," but even when tomorrow came, my attempts were fleeting—from hours to months.

Compassion began to replace my previous intolerance. I no longer saw noncompliant patients as disobedient hedonists, but as people struggling between hope and discouragement. And with this understanding came a new sense of responsibility. It didn't seem right to dish out advice without having lived the life I was advocating. I decided that for one month, I would live as though I had diabetes, complete with injections, blood glucose monitoring, meal planning, and foot care. I thought I knew what was involved; however, I soon learned that despite my years as a nurse, I really didn't have a clue.

The first time I plunged a needle into my abdomen was the only pleasant surprise of my tenure as a person with diabetes. Using a 30-gauge needle, my "insulin shots" (I used saline) were virtually painless. What I found painful was my constant vigilance surrounding my appetite. I could no longer eat what I wanted, when I wanted. I had to eat a half hour after each injection and again when the insulin peaked. I had to downsize my portions and decrease the amount of carbohydrates in my diet. I had to give up candy and potato chips, which took up too many of my carbohydrate choices. I'd always enjoyed food, but suddenly every meal was potentially fraught with guilt and shame, as I constantly struggled to make "good choices." I sorely missed my freedom with food.

What can I say about blood glucose monitoring? While it's a definite improvement since the days when patients had only vague symptoms and inexact urine dip sticks to guide them, it was one of the more challenging aspects of living with diabetes. It's more painful than insulin injections. It's also an intrusive and uncomfortable annoyance; one more reminder that life is no longer simple. Ordering, organizing, and toting supplies was a challenge. And I had the luxury of "adjusting to insulin" before I began monitoring. I can still only imagine the upheaval patients go through those first few weeks after they're sent home with a starter kit of insulin, syringes, lancets, strips, and lofty goals.

The first day, as I headed to lunch in the cafeteria, I realized that I had forgotten my meter in the office. I lost much of my break returning to retrieve my supplies. My original plan of testing four times a day was quickly replaced by a not-so-compliant once-daily schedule.

And then there was exercise. I love to walk, and when the weather is good, I normally walk up to an hour a day—but I never worry if I miss a day. But diabetes requires consistency, so I set a daily goal. Yet, every time I considered walking, I had to keep in mind my last insulin dose, when it was going to peak, and when I last ate. I had to remember to carry a source of carbohydrates in case I became hypo-glycemic. (I carried glucose tablets because I was afraid I would eat Lifesavers!) Again, the loss of spontaneity took the fun out of an activity I'd previously enjoyed.

As for foot care, I found I couldn't even remember not to walk in my bare feet, let alone check them every day. Those corns and calluses that threaten the limbs of those with diabetes remained just a minor annoyance to me.

I was often tempted to quit. But living as I was recommending became a very important exercise—one that fueled my desire to eliminate the word "noncompliance" from the medical vocabulary. My month with diabetes is now a starting point in my discussions with patients, who seem to greatly appreciate my efforts. And, now, I can fully appreciate theirs. ▼

The Pain

Susan's guilt.

Cortney Davis, MA, NP, RN

A young woman, whom I will call Susan, had been coming to our women's clinic for years complaining of intermittent deep pelvic ache that interfered with her sexual relationship with her husband. She'd had cultures for infection, Pap tests, ultrasounds—even an exploratory laparoscopy that discovered no adhesions, no cysts, nothing to explain her pain.

This particular day, she slouched on the exam table. Her short hair was blond and shining, but everything else about her was dulled. When I down, she met my gaze.

"Sorry I was late," she said. "But I just wasn't sure why I should bother to come."

"The nurse says that you're having pelvic pain," I said.

"Yes, but everything always comes back negative. My husband thinks this is all in my mind."

I hesitated a moment. "Do you think all in your mind? What do you think causes your pain?"

My question—had no one asked before?—released a torrent. Susan began to cry, lifting the sheet from the examination table and pressing it to her eyes. I thought I could guess the reason —rape or abuse, and my question somehow allowed her to acknowledge the pain. But Susan's story surprised me.

Susan told me she'd gotten pregnant at 16. She didn't tell her boyfriend, but she told his mother, who paid for Susan's abortion. She kept this secret from her parents and friends. Engaged, in her early 20s, she became pregnant again. Even though she wanted to keep this pregnancy, her fiancé didn't think the time was right; at his urging Susan had a second abortion, having felt forced to chose between his love and the pregnancy. Afterward, Susan became "angry and grouchy." Again, she told no one, ashamed that her fiancé had been able to convince her to end the pregnancy, an action that, deep down, she believed was wrong. They soon broke up, and for several years, every time Susan saw a child around the age her child would have been, she'd weep, alone. She even calculated when she would have delivered and, every year, spent that day crying. Five years ago, she married a "wonderful" man. She wanted to tell him about her two abortions, but the time never seemed right.

"After a year or so," Susan said, "he started to talk about our getting pregnant. That's when I started getting this pain. I don't think it's in my head. I think it's in my heart. What if I become pregnant and something goes wrong? How can I be a mother, after what I did?"

I had no answer. During my 17 years in women's health, I have seen women who have chosen abortion and have no regrets. I have also seen women hounded by unresolved emotion. Some are angry at the inadequate counseling. Some complain that caregivers minimized the procedure. Others report sudden remorse about an abortion they thought was "in the past." Susan mentioned two specific fears: She felt that she didn't deserve to be a mother, and she worried that any wanted pregnancy might be jinxed.

I have seen that it's difficult for some caregivers—those who assert that abortion is an elective procedure—to acknowledge that abortion can be a secret that weighs upon a woman's life like a stone. Susan was one of those women. She didn't need more tests. But how could I best help this woman whose life had been dramatically affected by the choices she'd made?

One way was by acknowledging that her remorse was real. Many women who have questions or regrets after abortion say nothing, believing that they are not supposed to feel anything other than relief. Trying to minimize or talk women out of their grief will only, I think, deepen feelings of guilt or shame. Susan told me that what she wanted most was to feel forgiven by God and to find a way to forgive herself.

Susan was depressed and anxious, particularly about telling her husband and accepting the idea that she deserved to become pregnant. Several weeks after our visit, Susan called to tell me that she and her husband were in counseling. She had found resources on the Internet. Slowly, she said, her physical and psychic pain was dissipating.

I am now, more than ever, sensitive to women who repeatedly seek help for symptoms when all tests are negative. Although I always inquire, I don't presume to know the answer. I ask women if they have *anything* in their past that might contribute to depression, grief, or guilt. Then I listen closely, not just to the words that play over the surface of a story, but to the message behind them as well. ▼

At the Night Camp

There's more to patients than their suffering.

Meg Sniderman, RN

Last summer I spent two weeks in South Georgia in my nursing school's Family Farm Worker Health Program. Involvement in the program fulfilled my community health class requirement, but that incentive didn't matter so much to me. The farm worker program was a chance to be among Latino immigrants, the population with whom I'd initially wanted to work, and to practice nursing in a new context: outside, under the open sky. My classmates and I stayed in Moultrie, Georgia, performing health screenings for the farm workers' children during the day and holding clinics for the workers every evening.

On the last night at camp I wasn't assigned to a particular station, so I served as an interpreter, filling in where needed. We'd set up camp in a dirt parking lot, and dust rose with our movements and settled on every surface like a fine gauze. We'd unrolled a tarp and laid out clothes for the workers, and as they came through they picked through the pieces, holding them up for size. Soon night fell, and people switched on their headlamps and walked looking down at the ground. Battery-powered lanterns sat on tables, but the only constant light came from the mobile pharmacy van, which glowed in the night.

The night passed quickly and as smoothly as any other, and when no more workers arrived and the intake stations sat empty, we began packing our equipment and breaking down the tables. A young man approached and asked if we could see him. He seemed timid but otherwise healthy. Since it was late, I wanted to be sure we could help him, so I asked him what kind of problem he had. "I need eyedrops," he told me.

Eye problems are common among field workers from exposure to sun, wind, and airborne debris; however, before he could see an NP, we had to check his blood pressure, glucose, and hemoglobin levels, and the equipment was already packed. We rushed to gather the supplies, and to speed up the process, I moved through the stations with him as his interpreter. When we reached the NP, she asked for his medical history and current problems, and while she charted his information, he and I talked.

He told me that he was 21 and had crossed the border from Mexico four years before, with his father's permission but without his mother's. I didn't ask if he had a visa. He said he had no family in the United States;

his five siblings still lived near his parents in Mexico. When I asked him why he'd come here, he said, "I guess I was bored as a teenager"—and then added, "I thought it would be different here."

The entire time he was with us he kept looking around, eyes darting back and forth and toward the truck he'd driven, which he told me wasn't his own. He shifted uneasily in his chair, and I felt the impulse to try to comfort him and tell him we could help. It wasn't an unreasonable thought, only foolish: though we may have held a loose authority in our makeshift clinic, he was able to navigate the surrounding area, and was more aware than we were of what it took to survive there.

I began to imagine what he might see: our blue scrubs and headlamps, our papers and instruments, all unfamiliar to him but superimposed against a land he knew intimately. After his consultation, he didn't want to stand out in the open, and he walked over to the truck to wait for his medications. I followed to make sure he didn't leave. Because he seemed so nervous, I asked if he had other questions or concerns he hadn't mentioned before. He looked at me very directly. "Yes," he said. I waited for more, thinking he might have held something back from the NP because they couldn't speak directly to one another. I steeled myself, expecting something difficult, but though he spoke earnestly, he said only, "I like you. You're pretty."

I smiled at him—and laughed at myself. I had made him into a tragic character, imposing hardship where I saw fit, but not seeing the whole picture. In certain ways he *was* a tragic figure—alone in this country, working long hours in poor conditions—but he was also a resilient human being, and to see only his suffering was to acknowledge only a part of him.

I saw then how easy it is to flatten our patients—to compress their personality into the framework of their needs. Those needs are never the whole story. ▼

Skipped Two Times

After a crisis, a dialysis nurse realizes her patients need more self-management education.

Shixiang Luo, MSN, RN

A young man in his early 20s, whom I will call Xiao Liu, had been coming to our department three times a week for several years for renal replacement therapy to help him discharge excess water and metabolic waste from his body. He was still in high school when he'd been diagnosed with renal failure as a result of systemic lupus erythematosus, and he never stopped studying, reading and writing, even during his appointments.

"I'm preparing for the university entrance exam," he often told me. He was upbeat and grateful, despite the disease. I admired him for his strength and spirit and felt terrible that he'd been diagnosed so young.

One day at 10 AM, the beeper rang, summoning the crisis team to the emergency unit. I hustled to the adjoining patient care tower. Mary, the charge nurse, told me that Xiao Liu needed a fistula puncture for continuous venovenous hemodiafiltration. He'd skipped his routine dialysis two times over the past five days; there was too much water and waste in his body, leading to acute left ventricular failure.

At the first sight of him—in high Fowler's position, coughing blood, pale with facies dolorosa, with pink frothy sputum on the nose and mouth—I felt brokenhearted. Breathing with difficulty, he said he was going to die and asked me to help him.

I waited for him to calm down and breathe more slowly as I prepared to puncture the fistula. The vascular pulsation was hard to feel, the murmur at the fistula too weak—obviously, his circulation had worsened. The blood flow was insufficient for extracorporeal circulation; the equipment alarm rang over and over. In this condition, he couldn't continue hemodiafiltration therapy.

Xiao Liu became agitated, shouting "I can't do it, I can't do it" and coughing bloody sputum more heavily. He grasped my hand in desperation, groaning, begging me to help him. Tears filled my eyes—although I wanted to help, there was nothing I could do but calm him down and instruct him to take deep breaths.

The emergency ICU physician arrived and immediately initiated emergency cannulation of a deep vein of the lower limbs. He soon achieved temporary vascular access for therapy.

After five minutes of therapy, Xiao Liu gradually began to resume his normal state. "Father said I was guilty," he told me. "I missed dialysis because I went to Beijing for a tour. This must be what I deserve. From now on, I'll never go anywhere else."

He began to weep, and for a moment I hesitated. Then I asked him, "Do you think yourself guilty? What do you think causes bad consequences?" In answer, he told me he'd looked up information about lupus on the Internet and thought he was going to die. Since his childhood he'd cherished two dreams—going to the Great Wall of China and going to college. In going to see the Great Wall, he'd wanted to realize at least the first of these before he died. Now, though, what he most wanted was to feel forgiven by God and to find a way to forgive himself. He seemed nearly overwhelmed with fear and unrest.

I patted him on the shoulder and nodded in response, assuring him that he could still have a long life, even with lupus and the need for dialysis. I had to see other patients, and I didn't come back until he was out of danger.

It's hard to put into words how ravaged Xiao Liu looked from his condition, his expression of pain, the telltale desperation in his eyes, and the sound of his pleading cries. He touched the heart of everyone who was there.

At the same time, I felt remorse at our department's weakness in patient self-management education, and knew we should put greater emphasis on how to control interdialysis weight gain from excess fluid in the future and tell dialysis patients not to miss regular appointments without permission. Despite the fact that they urinate little or not at all, many dialysis patients eat or drink as much as they did when they had healthy kidneys. If they don't get excess water and harmful solutes out of their blood promptly by dialysis, they can build up fluid in their lungs, heart, and limbs, resulting in discomfort or even sudden death.

Crises like the one that happened to Xiao Liu will keep happening if we don't do more to change patients' ideas and help them understand the importance of a healthy lifestyle. I now understand that it's my obligation and responsibility to help them with this. ▼

Tending Mr. Brown

She overcame the challenge, and then she met the person.

Dorothy Miller, RN

Valentine's Day at the senior center didn't seem promising. It had snowed the day before, causing the county to halt all bus service. Many of us had made it in only through the help of family and friends. As I sat with my cronies, I said to myself, "This is going to be one dull day."

Then the nursing students arrived. They checked blood pressure, discussed our medications, asked about our lives, and after much amiable conversation and banter, gave us a test to determine our mental acuity. They were young or almost young, and I was caught up in their enthusiasm. But I also knew they would have to master an ever-increasing array of skills and technology to meet the demands of today's nursing care. How many of them, I wondered, would go beyond those skills to become truly dedicated nurses? What would it take?

I remembered a time when I believed enthusiasm and skill were all I'd need in my career. In the 1970s, I was a staff nurse at the Lubin Rehabilitation Center at the Hospital of the Albert Einstein College of Medicine in the Bronx. Our unit was well known and respected throughout New York City. We cared for patients with all types of injuries and neurologic impairments, and I considered myself among the best of the nurses, minding neither the number of patients I was given nor how much care they required.

But there was one big flaw in my commitment. One type of neurologic impairment—Parkinson disease—so appalled me that I did my best to avoid patients who had it. It was a gut response. Maybe I just couldn't stand to be reminded of how helpless and vulnerable we all can become. (I'm still afraid of it: I'm visually impaired, and when I eat at a restaurant, I hate the idea that I could spill food on myself and not even know it.) This was more than 30 years ago, before patients with Parkinson disease were diagnosed early and treated with drugs to lessen and slow their symptoms. These patients were so rigid that it was a struggle to transfer them from bed to chair. They drooled, spoke in ghostlike whispers, had terrible tremors, and always wore their food at mealtime. I had made my feelings about this known to our team leaders, so I was never given these patients. None of my colleagues ever complained; they knew I could be depended upon to take difficult patients others might not be comfortable handling.

One day during the flu season we were short staffed. At the morning briefing, the team leader said, "Sorry, Dot, you'll have to take Mr. Brown today." I felt annoyed, alarmed, and challenged all at once, but I thought to myself, "I'll show them how to do it."

It was the practice on the unit to dress the patients in their own clothing, something we had long ago stopped doing with Mr. Brown. There were often food spills all over him, or a therapist would wheel him onto the unit soaked in his own urine. He would be put into his room to wait for his nurse, who was involved with the other patients' care.

In making out the care plan for my patients, I considered how I could find time to attend to Mr. Brown regularly throughout the day. I began by making the decision to dress him in his own clothes. After caring for each of my other patients, I retrieved Mr. Brown from wherever he was to get him to the toilet. At mealtime, I covered him with a sheet that caught all of his spills. After lunch, the patients sat around the nurses' station waiting to be picked up for their next therapy session. I was pleased when people passed by and said, "Mr. Brown, you look great today." He responded with a smile forced through the mask of his face.

I felt gratified by my success with Mr. Brown. I was settling him onto his bed for a rest before going off duty when I felt a tug at my uniform. I thought he had accidentally clutched it in the vise grip common to those with Parkinson disease. Turning to release myself, I saw that he was staring at me, trying to get my attention. I bent closer, and he said, in a whisper, "You ... don't ... know ... what ... you ... have ... done ... for ... me ... today."

Jolted by shame, I realized what really mattered—his dignity, his well-being. I hugged his rigid body and thanked him.

I am certain that there is a coming resurgence in nursing, part of the cycle of dying and rebirth that is in the nature of things. My wish for new nurses is that they might grasp what my teachers emphasized in nursing school a lifetime ago, but which I learned only from intimacy with patients: the importance of the three *Hs*—head, hands, heart—in treating the whole, sentient patient. ▼

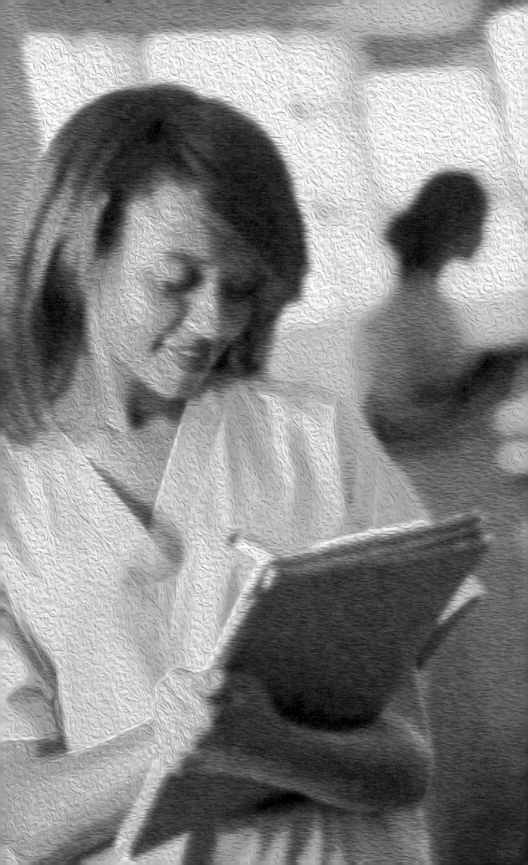

Getting Started

Stories by or about new nurses or nursing students—first
clinical experiences, patients that make a strong impression,
pressures from colleagues or preceptors, lives saved
or lost. Figuring out what really matters in nursing.

*"I don't think I'll be a good nurse. I know
I'll be a good nurse."*

Elizabeth Tillotson, BS

The Prospering of Cheaters

Revelaton in the NICU.

Ray Bingham, RNC

When they rolled the neonatal transporter carrying the very sick baby onto the unit, Marianne stood ready to admit him. As she carefully lifted him from the transporter onto the warming bed, the usual swarm of nurses, physicians, neonatal practitioners, and respiratory therapists gathered. At first, I stood far to the back. Only a few months out of orientation and still a nervous neophyte, I felt things went better when I stayed out of the way.

This time, however, I ventured close enough to watch. There was something I was curious about.

Marianne always seemed to take the new admissions and the complex cases. It wasn't so much that she volunteered, she just accepted the challenge. The charge nurse always sought her out.

Marianne was a southern belle—short, vivacious, with bobbed blond hair, bright blue eyes, and a warm, cheerleader smile. If you happened to be carrying a very sick baby down the street and you saw her, you wouldn't necessarily run to her first. In the NICU, though, she was tops: tough and smart and resolute.

That's what I was curious about. I believed in the nurse as a sort of comic book hero. Quiet. Decent. Defiant. Proudly independent—the Lone Ranger in scrubs and track shoes. I was determined to fly solo, but I kept getting grounded by reality. No matter how hard I tried, I could only do one thing at a time. I wanted to see how Marianne so deftly handled the barrage of demands in a crisis.

No sooner was the baby on the bed than the physician and the neonatal practitioner started barking orders for medications, drips, equipment, X-rays. They wanted to put in lines. They wanted everything *stat*. Marianne, in the eye of the storm, smiled calmly. She turned to Jo, "Could you mix my dopamine?" She turned to Irene, "Could you get the amp and gent?" She turned to Anne, the secretary, "Would you please call radiology?" At last she saw me, still lurking in the shadows, but not far enough removed. "Ray, could you bring a pump and make my UAC fluid?" I nodded. Who could resist that smile? But deep down I was angry. Hell, I thought to myself, I'm not learning a damn thing here. We're doing all the work. She's just staying at her patient's bedside, telling everyone else what to do. That's not nursing, that's cheating.

Gradually, I had a revelation: no nurse is a soloist. Once I accepted this, amazing things began to happen. One day I could use every spare minute of my time to help Laurie keep a baby off ECMO; the next, I could call on her to help me get an unstable cardiac admission to the cath lab. I could rush to the intermediate nursery to admit Sherry's baby who got septic; then, when I was confronting the parents with the overwhelming news, she could appear out of nowhere to help soften the blow.

I eventually became a nurse the charge nurse sought. She approached me one evening as I arrived at work. "Baby Angela might not make it through the night," she said. "Do you want to take her?"

Angela was the frailest of premature babies. I had admitted her a month before, when she hadn't been expected to make it out of the delivery room, and I had nursed her through the tenuous first days of her life. As fragile as she was, she radiated life to all who cared for her.

But her immature systems were beginning to fail under the onslaught of treatments. If this was to be her last night, I'd be honored to take her. However, Kim, a young nurse just months out of orientation, spoke up meekly in report. "I've had her two nights in a row. Would you mind if I took her back?"

"Of course not," I answered. "Just call me if you need me."

At two in the morning, the alarm went off. Angela's heart rate hovered in the 80s. She was dusky. Her oxygen saturation and blood pressure levels were sinking ever downward. We all rushed over. Someone brought the crash cart, and we started drawing up meds to prepare for the madhouse of a neonatal code. Then Kim tapped my shoulder. "Ray, the doctor wants me to start dopamine. Can you stay with Angela while I go to mix it?" Her voice trembled, and there was panic in her eyes.

She's afraid Angela's about to die. She's trying to back away so that I'll step in and take over. Deep down, I was angry. Damn it, that's not nursing, that's cheating.

"You're Angela's nurse, she needs you at her side," I snapped, and Kim startled at the sharpness of my tone. "I'll get the dopamine. That's what we're here for, to help you."

Angela survived that episode, although she hadn't long to live. Kim survived as well, looking stronger and more confident as we parted that morning.

Driving home, I pondered our propensity toward cheating. There are many ways to do it. Maybe you've just got to learn how to do it right. ▼

Touchy-Feely Stuff

Peace, love, and compassion in the hospital.

Sally Bellerose, RN

In 1977, while in nursing school, I was assigned to write an essay entitled "Inspiration, Aspiration, Vocation—Why I Want to Become a Nurse." This title suggested that motivations more lofty than mine were in favor at the school.

Job security and a living wage—not a burning desire to care for the sick—drew me to nursing. I was as compassionate as the next child of Woodstock, but to be honest, I would have chosen raising sheepdogs, becoming a folk singer, or being the girlfriend of a rock star first. If Jerry Garcia had shown any interest in me, I never would have gone to community college to become an RN.

At the time, I hadn't written an essay since I was in high school. I was working in the lingerie department at Sears and didn't see how my ability to make a guy feel comfortable selecting a night-gown for his wife was a skill I could use in nursing. So, as I sat cross-legged on my beanbag chair—every self-respecting former hippie owned one—I wrote about Anne, a hospital roommate from a few years earlier, when I'd undergone a total colectomy. While recuperating, my main pastime (besides watching television and pitying myself) was talking to Anne, who was afflicted by a wicked neurologic disease that made her twitch and jerk.

The only medical professional I saw respond appropriately to Anne's complaint of shoulder pain was a gray-haired nurse. She would perform her tasks—neuro check, blood pressure, meds—and fine-tune the bells and whistles on the medical machinery. Then she would fold her hands and ask Anne, "What do we need to do today?" She used the term "we" literally—meaning, how could they both make Anne more comfortable?

I watched her massage Anne's back and listened to their conversation, witnessing how she became Anne's trusted confidant and informed advocate. It looked so easy and natural. I wondered, "How hard can it be to focus for five minutes on the needs of a patient?" I was beholding the art of nursing. And with the grace of a skilled professional, Anne's nurse made it look simple.

In nursing school, however, I was overwhelmed by how much I didn't know. By that time, I had decided that the touchy-feely stuff was all well and good, but it seemed a luxury compared with learning the signs of diabetic shock.

But I sweated through that essay, piling on the sensitivity like the former flower child I was. I wrote what I thought would establish my potential as a nurse whose strength was exhibiting compassion. Consequently, the essay I turned in was not so much untrue as incomplete.

In nursing school, I decided to leave to the Dalai Lama the ability to stand still while holding chaos in the palm of the hand. But I could not entirely abandon the notion that someday I would become that nurse who calmed the tumult of the working day by folding her hands and listening to her patients. In the meantime, I strove to fill my frontal lobes with practical information that would get me through the next clinical trial. I had my eyes on the prize: I was going to graduate, pass the nursing boards, land a job, and buy a car that didn't require a screwdriver to shift gears.

One month after graduation and the day after test-driving a cherry-red Mustang, I found a job. On the first day, I faced a ward of 32 severely handicapped and developmentally disabled patients. I felt like an outsider, a frightened witness with pills to pass out, treatments to administer, and conditions to assess. Then I met the gaze of a 42-lb. woman named Daisy, whose small body was enfolded in a beanbag chair.

I knelt in front of her and attempted my first solo meds pass. She glared at me and clenched her teeth. I looked to the aide—"What do we do to get her to take the meds?"

"We say 'hello' before doing anything with Daisy," she replied. The aide grinned at Daisy and made a loud guttural sound. Daisy responded with a corresponding *"garr."*

"Hello, Daisy," I said, offering my own, tentative *"garr"*—but in too high a pitch. I repeated the aide's greeting until Daisy narrowed her eyes and gave me a near smile.

She took her meds, but the nebulizer treatment was another matter. I felt as though I were teetering on the edge of incompetence much of that day, but my gray-haired muse kept luring me back to solid ground. Sometimes I snarled at her saintlike image, but it always restored my composure when I interacted with patients. That weekend, I drove home a new Ford Escort. It wasn't as sexy as a Mustang, but it was cherry red and had a dynamite sound system that handled my tapes of the Dalai Lama and the Grateful Dead with equal ease. ▼

Where's My Hospice Moment?

An author's search for profundity in end-of-life care.

Lyssa Friedman RN, BSN, MPA and Coordinated by Veneta Masson, MA, RN

I sat in morning report, an eager new graduate on her first day on the pediatric oncology unit. I was ready to take on my dream job: administering comfort during the Ultimate Journey, holding hands with Those Who Stand at Life's Precipice. I'd already started IVs, and interpreted ECGs. Enough menial tasks, I thought. Give me Spiritual Nursing.

In my book I scribbled notes about my patients: Sam, a preschooler with leukemia, admitted for antibiotics. Kevin, a teenager with osteosarcoma and a below-the-knee amputation, scheduled for high-dose methotrexate.

"Time for rounds," my preceptor said, power-walking into Sam's room. "Vital signs. Intake and output." I scurried alongside. Check.

"Then we draw labs. White count. Type and cross. BUN. Creatinine." Check.

"Next we pass breakfast trays. Kevin will be too nauseous to eat."

"Baths, dressing changes," my mentor went on. "Hydration, antiemetics." How would I remember everything? By 8 AM my eagerness had turned to disappointment. Where were my hospice patients? Where was the hand-holding at the brink? My spiritual nursing practice?

By week's end Sam and Kevin had gone home, replaced by other young patients. I'd collected specimens, calculated drip rates, reviewed neutrophil counts, memorized side effects. I'd cradled a six-year-old who vomited, assisted in a lumbar puncture, restrained a three-year-old undergoing a bone marrow biopsy, and held the hand of a mother who couldn't believe her child had leukemia. I struggled to remember the significance of elevated liver enzyme tests; faces and facts danced in my dreams. And I forgot about providing spiritual care.

Then I settled on the evening shift. Mothers read stories to rooms full of bald preschoolers. Fathers met in the dayroom for cups of tea. When the single mom of a nauseated boy worked late, another mother wiped his face with a cold cloth and hummed lullabies.

Sam and Kevin came back for their monthly treatments, and their chemotherapy schedules coincided. Sam looked up to Kevin and often hung around the teenager's room. The little guy climbed aboard the bed and sat in the place where his older friend's lower leg had been. They played cards and watched television. Kevin gave Sam a San Francisco Giants cap on his fifth birthday. We rarely saw him without it. The rattier that hat became, the more attached to it Sam grew.

I enjoyed the long evenings after the charting was complete and the teeth were brushed.

One evening I toted Broviac dressing change supplies to Sam's room. Sam pulled off his shirt and settled back on the pillows, his Giants cap sliding off his head. His dad switched on the overhead light as I donned sterile gloves. Sam's tiny fingers loosened the tape around the two-inch square dressing.

I inspected for exudate, swabbed the exit site, applied a sterile dressing. I pulled off my gloves to rip strips of tape and affixed the 2-by-2 to Sam's chest.

"How old was Kevin when he had his leg cut off?" Sam asked.

"Sixteen. Why?" I said, gathering wrappers for the trash.

"How old will Kevin be when he dies?" I stopped my work and sat on the bed.

"I don't know. I hope he lives for a long time. Are you worried about Kevin?"

"I was just wondering how old I'll be when my leg gets cut off and when I die."

I felt the room start to tip. But Sam looked as though he'd asked whether he could have ice cream for dessert. His father watched him quietly, a weak smile on his lips. I explained to Sam that his diagnosis was different from Kevin's, that they received different medicines, that leukemia treatment did not involve amputation. By then a volunteer had wheeled a VCR into the room and popped in a videotape. Sam, distracted, jumped off the bed to sit in front of the TV.

I walked out to the nursing station. Sam's dad followed me.

"You know how some kids who are abused assume it's normal to be slapped?" he said. I nodded.

"Sam thinks it's normal to have a catheter sticking out of his chest. To be bald. To live part-time in a hospital. Kevin is Sam's role model."

Much later I realized that while I was holding out for my Hospice Moment—my moment in the presence of something profound—I had failed to notice the profundity all around me in the details of daily life. As I stripped Sam's bed, I untangled his baseball cap from the linens and handed it to him. The simple act of nonchalantly positioning it on his head revealed to me his acceptance of his illness and his future, whatever the outcome. Sam lived on the precipice every day. It was I who needed my hand held at the brink. ▼

My First Preceptor

A patient emergency alters the dynamic of a less-than-nurturing relationship.

Judith L. Reishtein, PhD, RN

"**M**anage your day," she told me, not for the first time, as if it had been my fault that one patient crashed yesterday just as my second one returned from surgery with a new set of orders. I could not be in two places at once, keeping track of two critical patients, making sure each one received the care she needed at the moment she needed it.

"Maybe you just don't belong in critical care," Doris continued. "You missed all your 10 o'clock medications and…"

I interrupted her. "At 10, I was at CT scan with Mrs. Smith—Janet promised she'd take care of Mrs. Ferrucci."

"She was your responsibility—you should have checked on her as soon as you returned to the unit."

My preceptor was supposed to help me adjust to the fast pace of critical care and guide me in the management of complex problems. But all she ever did was tell me the things I did inefficiently or wrong, that I could not keep up the pace, her tone implying that I was a disgrace to nursing.

She had been my preceptor since I started on the unit two months earlier, and as an experienced critical care nurse she had much to teach me. But she was a better nurse than teacher. Usually I just stood there, taking it all in, wishing I'd chosen another career, something less important, less vital, like growing petunias or polishing floors. But, perhaps inspired by the previous night's meeting at the high school about bullying, I fought back.

"I can't manage a day and neither can you," I said, a little too loudly. "No one can—we can only manage how we use the time we have. And I've done a better job with my patients and families this week than you have!"

I barely registered the shock on her face as I continued. "Both my patients required level 5 care, and despite that, I made time to talk to their families about what happened and why and what we're doing about it. How many families have ever thanked you when their loved ones died?" I had seen how annoyed she had been when Ed Smith thanked me for my thoughtfulness and support after we told him his mother had not survived her fifth cardiac arrest of the day.

"I'm doing my job," I pressed on, "and I'm doing it well, despite all your attempts to sabotage me. And if you'd just... "

My rant was interrupted by the alarm on the ventilator in Mrs. Ferrucci's room. We both raced in to see her husband standing by the bed, holding her hand, looking almost as panicked as she did as she struggled to breathe. "Sir, please leave," Doris commanded. "You're in our way."

He stood rooted to the floor, staring as the face of his wife of 63 years slowly turned from blue to gray. I squeezed his shoulder as I pushed past him and grabbed the Ambu bag from the wall. Tossing a suction kit to Doris, I said, "He can stay. He's not in my way."

Doris didn't say a word as she grimly tore the kit open. The noise was oppressive—now the heart monitor alarm had begun screaming, but I was too busy trying to force oxygen into Mrs. Ferrucci to reach over to the silence buttons. I couldn't compress the Ambu bag; her airway was completely blocked. Doris tried three times to insert the catheter and hit the blockage each time, but on the fourth try she managed to force through it.

And then, through all the alarm noise, we heard the thin squeak of air entering a partially cleared airway.

I reattached the Ambu bag and pushed a few breaths into her oxygen-starved lungs, and then Doris cleared more of the blockage. Both of us relaxed when we reattached the now silent ventilator.

Tears streamed down Mr. Ferrucci's face as his wife's face slowly regained its normal pale color. We straightened her in bed in silence, and then I turned to her husband before we left. "Can I bring you a cup of coffee?"

He looked up at me. "Yes, that would be good. And thank you," he said. He turned and looked across the bed at Doris. "Thank you both."

Doris accompanied me to the utility room and watched as I carefully poured his coffee and added two teaspoons of sugar and half an individual serving container of cream, the way I knew he liked it. As I picked up the cup, Doris spoke.

"You can react quickly when it's necessary," she said. "You did well in there. You'll be a good nurse someday." And she left the room.

I stared after her, repeating her words to myself. I'll be a good nurse someday. From Doris, those words meant the world. ▼

Bed Bath

The first day of the rest of my life.

Kathleen Hughes, MSN, RN, PNP-BC

Medical students start with cadaver dissection; nursing students start with bed baths. In preparation, I got the hair-washing cap from the supply room and warmed it in the microwave like a gas station burrito or a baby bottle. He wanted the basin water as hot as he could stand it, but I worried that my version of hot water might be more extreme than his. I brought in at least six washcloths and towels. There were many deep, quiet breaths.

And then the only thing to do was to begin. I started with his upper body, his chest. He leaned forward for me to wash his back. I draped him with towels as his hospital johnny got a little damp. I washed his legs and feet, and made a mental note to see if there were any nail clippers in the supply room, not yet having learned that nurses don't clip nails—whether because it's a billable service, or curiously dangerous, or simply too time consuming, I still don't know. He liked football, so I chatted about the Colts and Notre Dame, careful not to insult his Patriots or USC loyalty. His daughter was on another floor of the hospital birthing his first grandchild, so he turned on the newborn care channel. When he stood, not quite wobbly, to wash his own groin, I held up his gown and watched out for his IV and oxygen lines. Then I washed his bottom, donned him in clean hospital wear, and sat him in the chair. Last, I used the cap. As I massaged his scalp through it, and then dried and combed his hair, he sighed like I was a master masseuse or a magician who had cured his stubborn, inelastic lungs.

Should I describe his skin, his body, his face, so you can see him as I did? It was pale but not translucent, aged but not ancient, weathered but not beaten—and otherwise, I don't remember. Though I believed I would never forget his name, my first patient, it was gone from my mind within days, as if I'd internalized HIPAA rules as a command to forget, to deidentify. He had been a stranger to me when I arrived that morning, and if I bumped into him on the street a week later, he'd be a stranger again. In the moments of his exposure and my tending to him, his skin was both everyone's and his alone, as my hands were both mine and his.

Once he was clean and dry, I took another set of vitals, made some notes, got my lunch, and left the hospital—that intimidating and marvelous interior metropolis that I would like to call the Death Star for its massive, self-sufficient hive of wonder and industry, if not for the "death" part of the title. I have learned that the institution's preferred moniker, not entirely facetious, is Man's Greatest Hospital. Outside, it was blindingly bright, a cerulean October sky, and the old stones paving Beacon Hill seemed wise.

An Ivy League degree and 15 years of teaching and writing did not prepare me any better than my mostly 20-something counterparts in the ways of giving a bed bath to a 72-year-old man I'd never met. What might be different for me is that I have known many kinds of professional challenges. What might also be different is that I have lived enough longer to have attended my father's hospital-bound illness and death, and to have given birth to and cared for two young children. And so when I washed this man, I was washing my father, I was washing my children; I became one of those people who cared for us. Though giving a bed bath is not anything like lecturing to AP students on Faulkner, or writing a newspaper article on gun control or university library funding or modern exorcisms, I am not sure that either of those tasks made me hunker in a corner for five minutes, gathering myself before striding into the room. I've also never left a room feeling like I've had as simple and visceral an impact as I did that morning.

My work will get more technical and cerebral as I train toward my master's degree and NP certification, and yet my work will remain what it was that first day: bearing witness to the body in wellness and suffering, and honoring the dignity in that body, the dignity in the desire for the most basic of human care. ▼

A Nurse? What Was I Thinking?

The student's anxiety at starting a mentorship can feel overwhelming. Maybe that's all right.

Elizabeth Tillotson, BS

It's the night before the first day I will actually need to look like a nurse, the first day of my mentorship on the intermediate care unit.

I get my uniform all ready. I can hear mom's voice in my head: "Wrinkled clothes make you look less than you are."

Add "iron uniform" to checklist. Double-check list.

Lay out uniform. Pin name tag on, check with Significant Other to make sure it "looks straight."

Get stethoscope, hospital badge, and watch all laid out in one spot.

Double- and triple-check alarm so I don't oversleep. Make Significant Other do the same.

Midnight: Wake up… hope I don't oversleep.

2 AM: Why am I awake? Now I'll oversleep for sure.

2:15 AM: I guess it's OK to go to sleep…. I should sleep. I'll look tired and incompetent if I don't sleep. What am I doing? A nurse? *Really?*

3 AM: I'm screwed. I'm not sleeping. A nurse? Are you sure? No, I'm not sure, but I've already paid for the first semester—no turning back.

4:30 AM: I guess I slept some. But only one more hour and I have to get up. No, I shouldn't be a nurse.

5:30 AM: ALARM! I'm tired, I'm excited, I'm nuts. Yes, I *am* nut, *that's* it. It's just temporary, it will pass, please, please, let it pass.

I don the uniform. One look in the mirror: This is a long way from my business suit and heels. I take a deep breath. I've gone this far. I have to go one more day. I think, "This is a good thing!" This is a good thing? My mom's voice again: "Punctuation can change everything."

I report on time to my station. I present myself, lunch in hand, as confidently as I can. I'm greeted with smiles and warmth, and if I look really closely, a tinge of sympathy, which I accept.

My day is busy. I make mistakes. A half hour into the day, my mentor is showing me the electronic records system. "OK," she says, "now you log on and check our patients." I promptly click on the wrong program and launch software that will take 15 minutes to download. My mentor smiles and helps me click my way out of danger.

We are with a patient ready for discharge. Just one last check of vitals. My mentor instructs me to take the patient's BP. I think about the class lecture that week: patients judge you on how competent you are—especially if you're a student.

I try to put the cuff on as if I have done it a hundred times before. It barely fits. I check the size. I already have a large. I put it on and hit the button. The cuff begins to inflate. I hear the Velcro come to life as it strains to hold together under the increased pressure. Watching it grow, I'm terrified: Oh, please God, let it hold. I glance at the monitor: 160, 170, 180... the Velcro is angry, it doesn't care about me or God. It blows apart—taunting me, laughing at me as it slowly loses pressure, recoiling like a satisfied snake.

I apologize to the patient, tell her again that I'm learning. "That's OK," she says with a gentle smile, "we all make mistakes. I'm just glad I can help you learn. This isn't the first time that's happened." I put on my game face and try again, this time with success.

I realize my patient has just helped me learn, that she's attempting to take care of me and that maybe God did answer my desperate prayer. I failed at something, exposed myself—and in return, I got a smile, empathy, and encouragement from a total stranger.

The rest of the day is filled with hope for patients courageously fighting for a better state of health, and a profound admiration for those just fighting that fight because they still can.

When I go to bed that night, exhausted and depleted, I think of all the patients I had today. Are they OK? Did my blood pressure patient get to go home? Did the patient with kidney failure have a successful procedure?

I hope all of them are resting well.

What different thoughts I have in my head tonight. Just one last thought before I fall asleep:

I don't think I'll be a good nurse. I *know* I'll be a good nurse. ▼

A Special Kind of Knowledge

Learning what can't be taught in nursing school.

Janet L. Richards, BSN, RN

O n a Tuesday afternoon in 1973, during my second year of nursing school, I'm looking out the window on the eighth floor neurology wing, stalling for time. One of my patients from my rotation in the ICU has been transferred to the floor, and I've come to see her. Her name is Carrie. She's 20 years old and paralyzed.

I stood by Carrie during those first harrowing hours in the ICU as she awaited surgery, everyone still hoping for the best. As a brand-new student, I was a silent observer, unsure of how to participate. Her young husband also watched, slumped against the heater under the window at his wife's bedside. His eyes blazed, wild with fear and disbelief as he struggled to make sense of his sudden immersion into the alien world of disability. I could identify. Pressure sores, urinary catheters, bowel programs, and spasms—these were now part of my new and ever-expanding medical vocabulary. A spinal cord severed at C6 meant life as a quadriplegic. Suddenly this book knowledge seemed all too real.

At my post by the window on that day, I'm aware of my fear. I'm scared that the sadness and horror of what's happened to my patient will overwhelm us both. But I am a nurse and with grim resolve force myself to enter her room.

Carrie lies faceup and motionless, her passive body sandwiched between the two canvas slings of a narrow metal bed called a Stryker frame. A bag of amber liquid hangs along its side. Her hair is thick and long like mine, but a matted mess from weeks of neglect, her scalp still orange and crudely shaven at the temples where metal tongs pierce her skull to hold her head immobile.

I stand back as two attendants come to turn her. One stands at each end of the bed, counting to coordinate a quick flip. Carrie's body shifts slightly with the weight of gravity as the metal frame is turned. Overcome by the sensation of falling, and unable to exert any muscular resistance to alleviate her feeling of helpless passivity, she screams as she's rotated like an animal on a spit, the metal tongs tugging at her temples. One leaden arm falls, and she's powerless to stop it. My own scream is noiseless, caught in my throat.

Carrie is lying facedown now, with only time to spend studying the green and white squares of speckled linoleum beneath her face. I crouch on the floor by her head and look up. She smiles and greets me without a hint of sadness. "My husband's promised me a new wardrobe," she says, too quickly, "when I'm up and walking again. Mom's watching the kids."

She pines for her two young children and chats about their activities. She worries that her mother has more work than she can handle. She complains about the hospital food.

My mind scrambles for a reply. Thoughts of wardrobes, activities, and food float like helium balloons up to the tiled ceiling and then drift away. No response seems right.

When my silence finally breaks, I succumb to the very human urge to respond to another's pain by telling something of my own.

"I broke up with my boyfriend," I offer, regretting the words even as they fall.

For a moment we're both quiet. The air seems heavy. This was the wrong thing to say.

"Maybe you'll get back together," she says then, with flat hope, her face to the floor.

Our eyes meet in uneasy knowing. It's so apparent—we live in two different worlds.

Once again I've positioned myself by the window. It's evening and the cars on the street below have turned on their lights as commuters scurry home—everyone busy, full of plans, activities, and places to go, unaware of the suffering here. As much as I want it, there's no going back—no happy ending.

"I think I'm able to move my toes," she says.

Over four decades later, I still hear Carrie's voice and recall those words. I see myself at the foot of her bed, glancing out the windows with darkness closing in. I don't know it, but this is a pivotal moment as I force myself to turn toward her and look at the bottoms of her feet. Time loses meaning as I stand, head bowed, tentatively looking down at my patient's bare soles and frozen toes. I'm waiting, even hopeful.

Her feet aren't moving.

And then I know. Pain can be palpable as it moves across the space between two people, molten, unrelenting. Like joy and laughter, it's quite contagious. This is the special kind of knowledge I wanted, even craved going into nursing, and yet it's not at all what I expected. And this lesson will be repeated again and again and again.

Shared pain is still pain.

Some sadness will never let you go. ▼

Coming Home to Nursing

A new profession provides an unexpected sense of belonging.

Nancy Walters, RN

I had been taking care of people, in one way or another, for as long as I could remember, first growing up in Maine and then for 20 years in New York City. I had returned to my small town to help care for my mother, who had end-stage Parkinson's disease. After she died, I felt a void. I looked around at this tiny place, where people are considered to be "from away" even if they've lived here for multiple generations. I wondered what I had to give back to the supportive community I'd grown up a part of— and I also wondered if I could fit in after 20 years away. Could I turn my love of taking care of people, which I had always done outside of work, and make it my profession?

I was thrilled to be hired as a CNA as I worked my way through nursing school. My mother had passed away at one of the facilities where I worked, almost four years earlier. My first day on the floor, another aide and I were turning a somnolent patient, making her bed around her. The young CNA, eyes downcast shyly, quietly remarked, "We all miss your mother. She was a special lady." I was astounded. I had no idea that the staff would remember her—much less my connection.

Working as a nurse in the county where your family has lived for seven generations has a social complexity that can't be prepared for. In nursing school, my classmates had big plans: "I can't wait to move to Boston!" "I'm going to be a military flight nurse!" "My husband's job is moving him out West—I'll find a job wherever we go!" My only wish, which I kept to myself, was that I could work in my local hospital and never have to leave.

When I first saw the med–surg floor that would become my working home, I was one of a group of students. As we were handed our patient's information that first day, I was horrified to see that I had been assigned one of my grandmother's best—and most intimidating—friends from church as my total care patient. My teacher, sensing a learning experience, instructed me to ask the patient how she felt about my taking care of her. "I wouldn't want anyone else!" the patient exclaimed with a kind smile. I had never felt more proud, or more honored.

My place in the unit family progressed, from student and aide to new nurse. Faces became familiar. I realized how many patients value their ability to locate their caregivers as community members. I tried to imagine working in a large city, where patients would always be strangers. Some described their experiences "in the big hospitals" far away. An emaciated older man with throat cancer, who appeared to be alone in the world, returned to us after a procedure 100 miles south. He beckoned to me confidentially. I leaned over so that he could whisper. "I like it so much better here," he said softly. "You treat me like a real person."

Often, someone would see the name of a relative, a schoolmate, a family friend or ex-boyfriend on the morning's census and assignments were adjusted. I had thought I knew the community well, but the complex, surprising connections among people revealed how little I really had understood. I slowly realized that the entire community seemed to be related—to each other, to staff members, and also to me. "Why, you must be Barbara's daughter!" people I had never seen before exclaimed. Of course, they were right: I did look just like her. Once, a visiting daughter spoke into an elderly man's ear, "Did you know your nurse is Edith's daughter-in-law?" and turning to me, exclaimed, "She's so very proud of you!" I had never been sure what my mother-in-law thought of me. Now, a stranger was relaying her praise.

Familiarity with our patients spilled outside the hospital walls. A trip to the local Walmart or supermarket always seemed to include an interaction. I learned to assume that I had been everyone's nurse, or their family member's nurse, until proven otherwise. "Hi there!" a lady I couldn't quite place would say warmly, taking my hand, "Mom is doing much better now!" A middle-aged man in a camouflage coat smiled broadly as we waited in line at the deli and said, "I like seeing you out here better than in there!" "How're you doing, baby-doll?" said a jolly white-haired man with a nasal cannula in place, riding a scooter. He winked to my husband—who had no need to ask questions.

But more often than comments or updates, I would receive a silent nod of the head, or a shy private smile that I returned, both of us happy to be recognized for who we were: accepted, connected people in a small town, each fitting into our places. I became a nurse to give to my community. My community has given me so much more. ▼

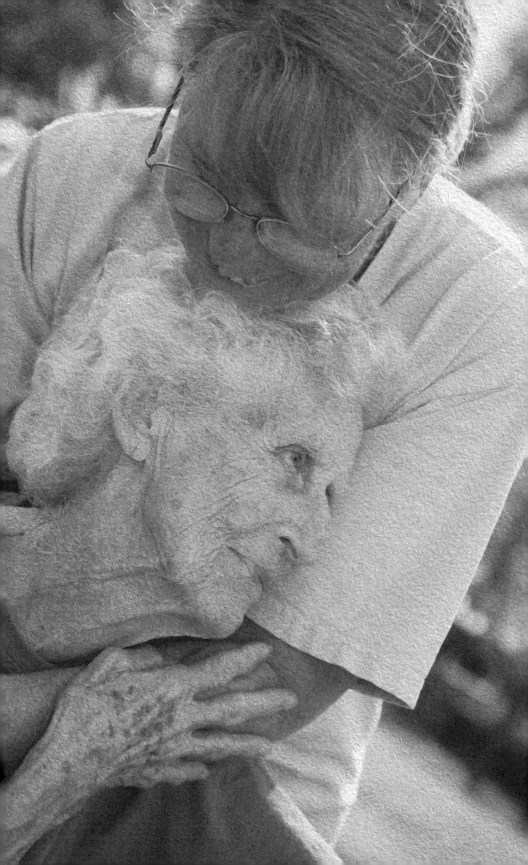

All in the Family

The roles of nurses in families—as mothers and daughters,
across generations, in weakness and in strength.

*"Given the choice, nurse or daughter, you
are always a daughter first – but the nurse
in you knows too much."*

Karen Schoonmaker, MSN, RN, CNL

Two Nurses—One Old, One New

A mother's example counts for a lot when the tables are turned.

Lois A. Gerber, MPH, RN

"Your mother has a brain tumor," Dr. Watts said.

My stomach flip-flopped.

"It's about the size of a small orange," he went on. "You're a nurse. You know the protocols."

Mom. A brain tumor? Always energetic and healthy, she'd been a little weak in recent months. But this?

I walked into her hospital room and found her alone. She was weeping. By the time our hug ended, her tears had stopped.

"Have you heard what's wrong?" she asked.

"No," I lied. I couldn't bear to say her diagnosis out loud.

"I have a brain tumor," she said, fingering the bedsheets. "Dr. Watts wants to operate."

I could only squeeze her hand.

She sighed. "It'll be all right. What's meant to be will be."

Like patterns in a child's kaleidoscope, the memories began to shift in and out. I remembered Mom caring for Grandma after the stroke paralyzed her. Mom ordered the equipment and remade Grandma's dining room into a sick room. She taught me how to bathe Grandma in bed, feed her so she wouldn't choke, and passively exercise her arms and legs.

But now Mom was in the hospital, unable to shower without assistance. Mom—the nurse so valued by her colleagues, the one who'd made nursing come alive for me since I was a child.

The next morning I carried a basin of water to her bedside to help her wash. As I wrapped the cloth around my fingers, I remembered how she let me splash my hands in the white enamel dishpan while she bathed my little brother. I was only four at the time and didn't realize that my brother was very ill. I watched Mom squeeze the red medicine into my brother's mouth from an eyedropper, and how she carefully peeled the tape from his skin, so slowly he didn't even flinch.

Now I was moving the washcloth down my mother's arm. She looked at me and smiled encouragingly, the way she did that day, while she bathed my little brother.

The nurse came in to give Mom her pills. Mom smiled as she took the medicine cup. I held the glass of water close to her chin so she could drink from the straw. When I was 13, Mom and my pharmacist father made me deliver medications to homebound seniors. I protested, not wanting to knock on strangers' doors. But Mom advised me to smile, ask how they were doing, and say something complimentary. Most of the older people smiled back; a few gave me cookies or candy. My interest in home health care—the very comfort I feel today when I enter a patient's home—is due in part to Mom's advice.

Later, as I was smoothing Mom's sheets, I remembered being nine and sick in bed with bronchitis. As Mom fussed over me, she told me stories about her patient, Robbie, a little boy whose leg had been broken in an automobile accident. She told me how he cried when she had to stick him with needles, and how she'd comfort him with a hug—and toast and jelly. "Grape was his favorite," Mom said, and that one little detail made an impression on me.

"Do you remember telling me about your patient, Robbie?" I asked, as I fluffed Mom's pillow.

"I do. He was a special kid. He loved his grape jelly." She smiled. "Sometimes the little things are what mean the most to patients."

And then I asked Mom how she felt about all her years in nursing, whether she ever regretted her choice of profession.

"Never," she answered. "Nursing has helped me understand what's important in life."

Dr. Watts had explained that there was a 50–50 chance the tumor would be malignant, but Mom seemed unfazed. "I've stopped worrying," she said. When I left the hospital the evening before the surgery, she appeared calm and upbeat. "I'll be fine, you'll see."

The next morning I arrived to find her lying on a cart in the hallway, looking so small and frail, so different from the day before. She raised her head and smiled at me. I kissed her cheek, but then the attendant came to wheel her into the operating room.

Hours later, Dr. Watts burst through the door of the waiting area in his wrinkled green scrubs. "We got the whole thing out," he said with a big smile. "It was benign, a meningioma. I don't anticipate problems. She's in recovery. You can see her shortly."

I sat by her side. Her head was swathed in a turban of white bandages. Her eyes fluttered open. "You're still here?" she murmured.

I squeezed her hand. "Of course."

"Two nurses, one old and the other new," she whispered, and fell back asleep. ▼

Morphine. Now.

Two sons, similar injuries—two very different experiences of pain.

Peggy Vincent, RN, CNM

"**D**islocated shoulder just walked in," the nurse had hollered. "I need 10 of morphine." My 24-year-old son Colin had just lurched into the ED of a private hospital on California's coast after a weightlifting mishap. "Allergic to anything?" the nurse had asked. When Colin had said no, she'd immediately injected morphine, saying, "With dislocations, we have a standing order. Morphine first; questions later."

When I arrived 15 minutes later, Colin was calm and blessedly woozy. But he held his arm at a strange angle, and I couldn't stop staring at the sickening hollow where his shoulder should have been.

I was grateful that my son was made comfortable while waiting for treatment, especially with something as painful as a dislocated shoulder. As a former delivery room nurse, there were times when my first response upon a woman's admission was to obtain an order for pain relief. I remember thinking as I kissed my son's forehead, "This is how it should always be."

Four years later, my other son, Skylar, an athletic 15-year-old, arrived at the ED of the largest HMO in the San Francisco Bay Area. He had blocked a shot during a pick-up basketball game and dislocated his shoulder. His screams silenced the crowded waiting room, and he held his arm at that same, familiar, stomach-turning angle.

I know how hospitals function. I know the right language, how to work the system, but none of my 35 years of experience helped my son. I said to a physician, "You're a doctor, right? We need an order for pain medication. Please make my son comfortable while he's waiting." Nothing happened.

A nurse started an IV and left. I approached an ED guard, a registration clerk, a triage nurse, an ED orderly, five nurses, and two physicians. I appealed to them as an assertive nurse and a desperate mother. Nothing worked. For 90 minutes people in white walked past us and did nothing except offer meaningless updates: "We've called the ortho doctor," or "We'll give him something as soon as we have an order." For 90 minutes my demands and pleas produced no one who said, "Morphine. Now."

As a nurse and midwife, I was usually able to provide relief with my presence and speech, my touch, or merely by making eye contact. But when my patients needed pain medication, I was forceful in getting a doctor's order—immediately.

But standing beside my writhing son, I marveled at the callous attitude of most of the employees. How would they have responded, I wondered, if this screaming teenager had been their child?

At last a nurse came and stayed. She called Skylar by name, started oxygen, requested an X-ray, and treated me like a colleague. But without a doctor's order, she was as helpless as I was to ease Skylar's pain. Three times she called the orthopedist to request pain medication, but each time she was told, "He's not available." She confided that, because of her dissatisfaction with this HMO, she was quitting in two weeks to work at a private hospital.

Eventually the orthopedist arrived, an expressionless man with the bedside manner of a bottle of saline. He didn't acknowledge me, nor did he respond when spoken to. He ordered morphine and left without speaking. The nurse injected the drug immediately.

"Wow, my brain is clogged. That's so weird," Skylar said, but 10 minutes later he moaned, "It's not enough," and again his screams rang through the corridors.

When the doctor returned, I said, with forced composure, "He wants to know if he can have more."

"We're taking care of him," he said in a monotone.

Yeah, right, I thought.

Skylar received a second dose and finally fell asleep. For the first time in 90 minutes, I relaxed. Ten minutes later, the poker-faced doctor did an adequate reduction, straightened his lab coat, and disappeared. We never saw him again.

Like his older brother's, Skylar's shoulder injury healed well. But their experiences in the ED couldn't have been more different. One got morphine sooner; the other got it later—and suffered horribly. Since then, I've tried to fathom the possible causes of the differences in their treatments. Regardless, I know my youngest child suffered far too long.

These two experiences reinforced my belief that nurses need more autonomy in providing pain relief. While my midwifery patients rarely asked for pain relief, my ability to provide immediate relief when requested was one of my satisfactions—I didn't have to wait for a doctor. I had standing orders signed by a physician under whom I practiced, and those orders gave me wide latitude. Why don't ED nurses have the same independence? ▼

At the Eye of the Storm

A nurse struggles with medical decision making for her ailing father.

Karen Schoonmaker, MSN, RN, CNL

The priest was the first person I saw as I rounded the corner and entered the ED. *It must be all over*, I thought. *He's already gone.* I rushed in and laid my head on my dad's chest; something hard met my cheek. It was an ECG lead. I remember feeling so confused about that hard nub. I was relieved he was still alive. I looked toward my mother sitting off to the side. She looked at me knowingly, as if resigned.

She'd called me two hours before. My father had collapsed at their home. He'd spent the previous week preparing for Hurricane Earl, boarding up windows and tying down boats. In the two hours since the call, things had gone from bad to worse. At the hospital, he was quickly intubated and ultimately transferred to the ICU. He'd had a large MI, was in pulmonary edema, and his body was shutting down.

That night, as the hurricane blew up the coast, our family sat huddled in a storm of our own. We took turns sitting in the corner of his ICU room. Dad was sedated and intubated. The monitors showed blood pressures that were much too low. He required large doses of medication to sustain his blood pressure. His nurse moved purposefully from monitor, to IV pump, to ventilator, back and forth. Throughout the night she never sat down, pausing to speak with us only briefly to offer support, to offer short explanations, or to give my mother a blanket.

In hushed tones, my mother and I discussed how sick my father appeared. We understood a hard conversation and a difficult decision were imminent. Things looked so bleak we were sure we would have to let him go.

Early the next morning, we gathered for a family meeting with the physician. I realized my siblings and I are not so rare. As we became adults, we became more distant. We were joined together by a dying parent, about to make a life-and-death decision.

The physician shared the plan—a cardiac catheterization and an intraaortic balloon pump were needed. A cardiac surgery might well follow. Since contrast dye was required, my dad's already failing kidneys might be further damaged and dialysis could become necessary.

The gravity of the situation was paralyzing. We spoke with the physician, weighing comfort measures over treatment. We spoke about how to proceed. My mother and I, both of whom were nurses, felt compelled to describe what the overall state of his health might be if he were to survive his hospitalization and what type of care he might then need to make a recovery. We all knew he was a proud and strong man. Was this the kind of life he'd want?

Then I remembered a brief conversation I'd once had with my dad. I'd asked him if he wanted everything done, and he had replied emphatically that yes, he did. During the family meeting, I retold this story. It galvanized our family. We realized that despite the horrible odds, this is what he would have wanted. Once we'd made the decision, we felt as if we'd been thrust onto a path with an uncertain destination for both our father and ourselves. We were fairly certain that his chances for survival were slim, and even less so for a full recovery.

As we got up to leave the room, my father's nurse emerged from the background. I felt her arm around my shoulder. "You're doing the right thing," she said gently. I didn't believe her, but I was relieved to have the decision made and to have respected my father's wishes.

Nothing can prepare you for having a critically ill parent. Given the choice, nurse or daughter, you are always a daughter first—but the nurse in you knows too much. It is a bit of a curse. I knew my father wanted everything done, but I didn't know if in choosing everything he'd realized what that meant. Neither choice was clear; the absence of an advance directive made decision making even more challenging.

It's been a year since that family meeting. Another storm threatens to batter our coastal town, this time Hurricane Irene. I am outside the cottage battening things down. As the wind picks up, I remember how I felt a year ago, the unbelievable circumstances I found myself in. Like many other families with a sick loved one, we were faced with nearly impossible decisions. Did we do the right thing?

I see an old red truck approaching the house; behind the steering wheel is my dad, and he smiles with delight. He has come to make sure we board up the house in preparation for the latest storm. ▼

Census of One, Staff of Five

A family of nurses gathers to care for one of its own.

Elizabeth Corso Falter, RN, CNAA, BC

C arol and I decided: our sister Sheila needed to be moved from the sofa to a hospital bed in the living room. Sheila shook her finger at me and said, "No"; she knew too well what a hospital bed in the living room signified—sick people who weren't dying rested on the sofa. But I insisted, and she let us move her. I tried to ease the transition by playing a CD of Civil War tunes. Sheila tapped her bony knees to "Battle Hymn of the Republic," as I rolled her wheelchair across the room.

Sheila, a registered nurse for 35 years, was dying of pancreatic cancer. My sister Carol and I, nurses with more than 30 years' experience each, knew the perils of pancreatic cancer, and we knew that we had to go to her right away. We met one day at Sheila's house in Maryland to help her husband take care of her. After a few days, Carol and I decided to give Sheila's husband and caregivers a break, and we sent for the other nurses in our family. My nieces Rita and Anne Marie represented the second generation of Corso nurses, and they were thrilled to come.

That clear, warm night in June my sister Sheila became a census of one with a staff of four nurses—Elizabeth Corso Falter, RN; Carol Corso Bodine, RN; Rita Bodine Meadows, RN; Anne Marie Corso, RN—plus my daughter Carol, my sister's namesake. Our hospital consisted of Sheila in the living room, our sleeping quarters in the adjoining recreation room, and our nurses' station in the kitchen. The patient, who felt better because fluid had been drained from her lungs, decided to take charge. First, there was a birthday to celebrate; my daughter Carol turned 25 that day. Sheila had ordered Rita, the baker, to make a cake to surprise Carol. Rita arrived with a white cake with blue icing trim and decorated with items from her children's parties—candles, plastic balloons, clowns, turtles, and Power Rangers—25 items in total. That cake looked like it had been made at two hours' notice, but we savored it.

Sheila appointed my sister supervisor and me hospital administrator. We went to the kitchen to devise a nursing care plan. Our diagnoses were standard: alteration in skin integrity, pain, fluid volume deficit, and alteration in respiratory status. Our care plan included full-body massage using balms Anne Marie had brought. Sheila suffered from pruritus, especially on her buttocks. As Anne Marie or Rita massaged Sheila's back, starting at the shoulders, Sheila instructed them to go lower and lower; the plan came to include what Sheila called "butt duty."

It was midnight when I reviewed our plan with Sheila and the full staff. After the brief review, Sheila—forever directing—told me I could go to bed. As I drifted off in the recreation room, I heard the sounds of nurses carrying out their duties: the rustle of sheets as Sheila was turned, whispers about pain medication: "she won't take it," "afraid to sleep."

Later that night, Sheila told our sister Carol that she didn't want to die. Carol felt unprepared to receive this confidence, searched for a response, and remembered a rainy night when Sheila was eight and Carol 10. Sheila had had a bad dream and Carol woke her, drew her into a hug, and said, "It'll be okay." Now, decades later, how was one to respond to this very real nightmare? Carol hugged her, as she had when they were children. "I will do everything I can to help you live," she said. "But if I don't succeed, Dad will be waiting for you." Sheila said, "Okay," and then let herself fall asleep while Carol watched over her.

At 6 AM I got up to check on our patient. I noticed that Carol had crawled into bed with me during the night. When I entered the living room I saw Sheila, awake in her bed. She raised her finger to her mouth to shush me. Rita lay on the sofa, my daughter Carol in a chair, and Anne Marie across the bottom of Sheila's bed. Sheila had been awake for hours while the entire night shift slept.

Her health improved, briefly, after that night. She ate more and even took short car trips. Sheila's staff of five went back home, and her husband and other local family took over her care. She died in September. But during that night in June, we were able to deepen our already strong bonds as sisters, aunts, nieces, cousins, daughters, women, friends, and nurses—and for that we who remain are all grateful.

So the next time someone asks me about the best staffing conditions, I'll tell them: a census of one and a staff of five. Midnight shift. A beautiful night in June. ▼

A Nurse's Mother's Nurses

The RN, the CNA, the LPN ... she needed them all.

Donna Diers, PhD, RN, FAAN

They walk toward me in the cemetery in a little town in Wyoming where we have just buried my mother: Linda, Carol, and Beverly, my mother's nurses.

Mom's osteoporosis had shrunk her from her proud 5'4" to barely 5'. Arthritis had turned her hands into claws. Chronic obstructive pulmonary disease, which tethered her to an oxygen machine hidden discreetly behind a living room chair, had caused congestive heart failure. She was on enough medicines to fill the biggest plastic container the drug store carried.

I lived many guilty miles away in New England and my brother was a full day's drive south in Colorado. Dad took care of Mom and it had become a full-time job. The only time he really got away was just after dawn, while Mom was still asleep. He would meet an old friend for a quick round of golf on the rough public course where the fairways were sagebrush and weeds and the greens were beige sand.

Mom and Dad decided they needed a little more help at home. I was relieved when I heard that community health nurses—my professional sisters—were going to be involved.

Carol came first. She was an LPN. Deeply tanned, she looked as if she'd be more comfortable on a horse than in her Subaru and spoke only when she had something important to say. Carol took over the complicated medication regimen and the weekly "checkin' in."

Not long after, Linda joined the team. Linda was a nursing assistant. The flaming red hair I remembered from when she was growing up a few years behind me had faded to dusky rose. Linda came two or three times a week to help Mom with her bath, a task that had Dad buffaloed. Mom and Linda clicked right away, and when I was there on one of my increasingly frequent visits, Mom would rather have Linda help her. I would listen to them laugh as Linda jollied Mom through the shower that exhausted her. She was especially good with Mom's hair, about which she was deservedly vain. Hair care has always escaped me.

Mom began to slip a little bit more every time I flew in.

Without telling Mom and Dad, I went to the community health agency to see Beverly, an RN and case manager. I needed to sort out how to talk to my parents and shore them up. Bev, a calm, centered woman with huge brown eyes, suggested that we all meet. When we did, and we sidled up to the question of palliative care, Mom refused to be dying.

Then one day Mom got breathless and Dad took her to the hospital. The X-ray showed lung cancer. When Mom told me about it on the phone as I was preparing to visit them, she seemed almost relieved. As a long-time smoker, she understood getting lung cancer. Although it probably wouldn't do much more than relieve her labored breathing, radiation was planned, in keeping with Mom's desire to be treated. Dad was tired and anxious about what might be next. We decided that short-term nursing home placement just up the street from their home would be best. Mom agreed.

I wanted her there too, in the hands of nurses—she already knew many of them, since her own mother had been a patient there, as had many of her friends. I helped with the move. Knowing I had a professional commitment in Arizona, I had packed my fancy dress. Mom loved clothes, so I modeled it for her in the nursing home. She liked it. She even said my hair looked good.

But Mom didn't settle in. She got twitchy and irritable. She began to call Dad at dawn, at noon. Dad started going to the nursing home early in the morning and spending most of the day with her. When I returned home from Arizona, the RN in the nursing home called and we had a conversation that led to a tricky dialogue with mom's physician about using morphine to make her more comfortable.

I got on a plane again.

Carol came to visit Mom in the nursing home. Dad was there. Mom was sleeping but woke to Carol's voice, smiled into the middle distance, took a deep breath, and died. I was somewhere over Iowa.

It took a small squad of all kinds of nurses to care for all of us.

Now, at the cemetery, I hug Linda, Carol, and Bev—a CNA, an LPN, and an RN—in wet, salty gratitude. They did for my mother what this fully credentialed, multiple degree–bearing nurse daughter couldn't do. They made all the difference to her—and to me. ▼

A Place for Palliative Care

Families have a right to know the true meaning of 'survival.'

Carrie A. Bennett, MS, CNS-BC

I haven't seen her yet, but my husband has been updating me on her condition. He doesn't understand medical terminology, and his updates have lost some detail in translation, but I'm able to piece together a story that sounds logical: my mother-in-law's condition is grave. The chemotherapies used to put her leukemia into remission have savaged her body, and she doesn't have the reserve to fight this new respiratory infection. I don't know how to tell him this, so I just hold him and say that we should go and be with her. I'm a nurse, but I'm also his wife.

When I do see her, she looks just as I'd envisioned. She is sedated and intubated. The monitor above her bed shows a blood pressure of 68/46, a heart rate of 174. I expect to hear a critical alarm, but the monitor has been silenced. Her face is flushed, and her extremities are cool. She is on vasopressors and antiarrhythmics. She is on antibiotics, antifungals, and antivirals. A continuous renal replacement therapy machine sits beside her bed, waiting to dialyze her, but her pressures are too low. She is third spacing. I subtly pull the white sheet up to hide the fluid weeping from her extremities—something her children don't need to see.

Physicians say she has a chance of surviving with continued aggressive treatment. She is a "full code." Family gathers around her, holding onto the chance, misinterpreting survival as recovery. I don't know how to tell them the difference, so I stand aside. I'm a nurse, but I'm also their in-law.

A family meeting is called and I'm invited to attend. Physicians tell the family that her lungs are damaged, her liver is damaged, her kidneys are damaged, and her heart is damaged. They don't know how her brain is doing, but think it may be damaged as well. They reiterate the chance of survival and answer the one question I'd posed to them earlier: would a palliative care consultation be appropriate at this point? "No," they tell us, "she can still survive." Her family agrees to pursue aggressive care. She would want to survive, they reason. But survival continues to be mistaken for recovery, and no health care provider has explained otherwise. The physicians excuse themselves to insert a line in her femoral artery. I sit with the family. I'm their in-law, but I'm also a nurse.

I'm a nurse with years of experience in palliative care. Years of encountering similar situations: families caught up in a reality created by a misunderstanding of the medical world and its language. I carefully open up discussion and hold the palliative care consultation the family so desperately needs. We talk about the implications of her damaged organ systems—chronic ventilator support, dialysis, artificial nutrition—the likelihood of brain damage. We talk about her definition of quality of life—traveling the country with her beloved husband, hosting grand holiday gatherings, and reading to her dear, sweet grandbabies. And in our discussion it becomes apparent that she wouldn't be satisfied with simply surviving. She would want to recover—an unlikely feat at this point in her illness.

The physicians are updated and her code status is changed. Family gathers around her bedside and she dies a short while later. They're sad but appear at peace with their decision to let her die with dignity. The physicians gather around her bedside too, offering condolences. Their demeanor is professional, but they appear defeated—an ICU patient they couldn't save. I'm sad for all of them, including the physicians.

The finality of death is a concept so difficult to grasp. And, somehow, the medical culture has come to equate the finality of death with the ultimate failure—a detrimental view that precludes acceptance of palliative care services into most intensive care settings. My mother-in-law's death was not a failure, but rather an outcome of our attempt to respect her wish to *live*, not merely survive. Failure would have been to keep her alive, chronically dependent on a ventilator and dialysis and fed through a tube. ▼

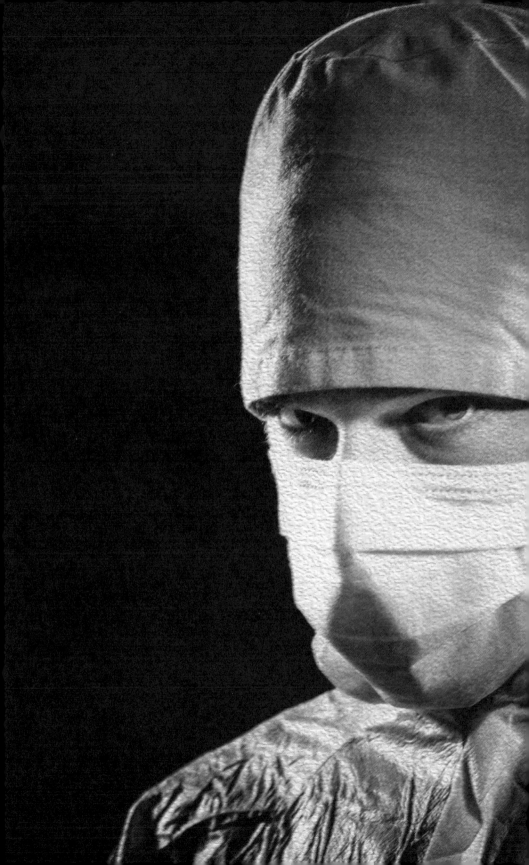

Doctor Jekyll and Doctor Hyde

Nurse–doctor relationships and the related questions of respect, power, and experience vs. clinical/professional status. Reversals, resentments, gratitude, team work.

"And I have remained indebted to that nameless nurse of the night ever since. And to so many others throughout my career who quietly saved me."

Michael M. Bloomfield, MD

Last Rights

A wedding in the ICU.

John A. Forrant, BSN, RN, CCRN

At his morning assessment, Mr. Casal (not his real name) didn't seem like the man I had met 24 hours earlier. Yesterday he'd been full of life, talking with staff and family members, laughing at my attempts to say "hello" and "how are you?" in Spanish. This morning he sat bolt upright, his breath rapid and shallow, his color ashen. I held his cold hands in mine and asked how he was doing. "Not good," he said.

Mr. Casal had end-stage pulmonary fibrosis, and I was convinced he'd soon need to be intubated and placed on a mechanical ventilator. After discussing this likelihood with the resident, I shared my concern with Mr. Casal and his daughter (he understood and spoke basic English, but she translated when necessary). They spoke together for a few moments, and then she told me her father didn't want to be intubated.

She asked whether we'd give her father morphine to keep him comfortable. I asked the resident to call the attend-ing physician. He did so, and was given an order for a single dose of morphine 2 mg IV, which I then administered.

I'd been struck by the joy Mr. Casal and his family seemed to take in one another's presence. Now my primary concern was to keep him com-fortable and to make sure he'd be able to interact with them for as long as possible. I returned to the hallway to speak with his daughter. With tears in her eyes, she told me that she was getting married in a month and that one of her father's greatest wishes was to see her married. I suggested I call our chaplain to see if we could arrange a wedding on the unit.

While Mr. Casal's daughter hurriedly called her fiancé and asked him to come to the hospital with the marriage license and rings, I called the director of pastoral care, who agreed to the plan and put in a call to one of the chaplains.

When the chaplain arrived, he advised the bride and groom to be pre-pared for a celebration that would almost certainly cause mixed emotions. The groom replied that he frequently had dreams involving his "guardian angel" and that this morning his angel had visited him and instructed him to go see his future father-in-law in the hospital and to bring the rings.

Before we could conduct the wedding, the attending physician arrived. He berated the resident and me for what he perceived as a breach of protocol in our addressing end-of-life issues without his permission. I felt dread in the pit of my stomach as I listened, but I didn't believe I'd done anything more than respond to the concerns of a patient and his family.

I reminded the physician that he was required to address the patient's stated preference not to be intubated, but he angrily told me that before we could conduct the ceremony he wanted to make sure Mr. Casal had been offered "every possible" option, including intubation and transfer to a facility that offered additional treatments. During the subsequent conversation with Mr. Casal and his family, the physician kept saying "we would have to breathe for you," but never mentioned intubation and long-term ventilator support. When I explained to the family that the physician meant a breathing tube would have to be inserted, they all looked at me in horror, and the patient again refused intubation.

The physician wrote out a "care and comfort" order for Mr. Casal that included morphine and sedatives to be given as needed. As we left the room, he rebuked me for speaking up, but I told him I had only been trying to clarify his thoughts.

Shortly afterward the chaplain entered the room in his white robe and purple stole. He was newly ordained, and this was his first wedding ceremony. All thoughts of code status and vital signs disappeared as about 20 hastily gathered family members surrounded Mr. Casal's bedside. Feelings of warmth and acceptance filled the room.

Throughout the ceremony a baby slept quietly on Mr. Casal's bed. When the minister asked, "Who gives this woman to be with this man in the sacred covenant of marriage?" Mr. Casal raised his arms, grabbed the hands of the bride and the groom, and declared: "I do. I am her father!" The groom promised Mr. Casal that he would always take care of his new wife.

Afterward, as the family mingled around a small cake, Mr. Casal's daughter, crying, gave me a big hug and told me I was her guardian angel. Mr. Casal died quietly with his family at his side within 16 hours of the wedding. ▼

My Turn

A retired physician recalls how a nurse helped him out of a predicament as a new intern.

Michael M. Bloomfield, MD

Medicine was my first rotation as an intern. At University Hospitals of Cleveland, the medicine rotation had a particularly intimidating reputation and a red-hot I was not. I was terrified.

On morning rounds every day our entourage of physicians, nurses, and students would go room to room discussing each patient. I can still see the open door to Mrs. Finkelstein's room near the morning sunlight at the end of the hallway. Mrs. Finkelstein was old and was dying. And every morning when we walked in, her husband was sitting there next to the bed, holding her hand. He told us regularly how many years they had been together. We each dreaded being the one on call when she died.

Call was every third night and was grueling. One night when it was my turn, my senior resident pulled me aside after sign-out rounds and said that Mrs. Finkelstein would probably die on my shift. I wasn't ready. In medical school they taught us everything about keeping someone alive, but no one ever told me what to do when a patient dies. I had never pronounced a patient dead before. No one had even explained to me how to tell if someone is dead.

He could tell. He said take your time. Be respectful. Be methodical. Be confident. Appreciate the meaning of the moment for the family. Listen to the heart, look for respiratory effort. Talk straight. Stay for as long as the family needs you. And then he left me in charge of the floor for the night.

Call was mayhem. Always. The night was spent frantically admitting patients, taking histories, doing physical exams, checking labs, writing orders, starting ivs, talking to family members, flaming broth tubes for blood cultures, doing manual white cell differentials, and the 10,000 other things that an intern had to do in those days on a medicine rotation at University Hospitals of Cleveland preparing for the assault at morning rounds. Sleep was never really an option.

Somewhere in the middle of the night and the chaos a nurse came up to me with that look, and I knew. I wasn't ready. She could tell. She came with me.

He was there, holding her hand as always, eyes wide. His whole world depended on me. I walked in quietly, looked for respiration and listened to her heart for a long time. Nothing. I took the stethoscope out of my ears and looked at him with genuine compassion and said, "I'm so sorry." He looked down at the bed, dazed, and we stood there in silence, sharing the weight of the moment.

That's when it happened. Mrs. Finkelstein breathed an enormous sigh! We all froze. I was mortified. Mr. Finklestein looked at her—looked at me—looked at her—looked at me.

"What was *that*?!" he said. I tried to look calm. "Well, is she dead or isn't she?" he yelled. Inside, I was reeling. *What the hell? Is she dead or isn't she? Four years of medical school and I can't tell if someone's dead?!* Time froze—the moment remains suspended in my memory still. I don't know how long we stood there, but it felt like such a long time.

"After a person dies there are last gasps," the nurse explained to him quietly as if it came from both of us. "Not unusual." I nodded authoritative agreement, expressed my deepest condolences, stayed as long as I possibly could, and went back to the 10,000 things. And I have remained indebted to that nameless nurse of the night ever since. And to so many others throughout my career who quietly saved me. ▼

A Smart Doctor Listens to the Nurses

A pediatrician pays tribute to her mother's career.

Ann Fleming Beach, MD

I was in the hall outside a patient's room with a new crop of interns and residents. As usual, they had all made rounds first thing in the morning, checked on new lab results, examined their patients, and were now ready to report everything to me, the attending. And, as usual, these bright, eager residents, though anxious to do a good job, hadn't thought to talk with the nurses taking care of their patients.

I patiently started my spiel. "You dart in and dart out. Your impression of your patient is like a snapshot. Your patient's nurse has been here for 12 hours. Her impression is like a video. You can't tell me you've made rounds unless you can tell me the nurse's name and what she has to say." I continued, "Say this to the nurse, each time: How are things? Anything you're concerned about? Anything you think I should know? Any orders you think I might want to change?"

My residents seemed surprised by this notion. I called the nurse Susan over. She told us the grandmother of one of our pediatric patients had unexpectedly died the night before, so the parents were anxious for discharge so that they could mourn and arrange the funeral. She also suggested we could stop IV fluids, since the child had just had a good breakfast.

This was all news to the residents.

I'm the daughter of a nurse. When I went off to medical school, Mom told me, "I don't often give unasked-for advice. But I will tell you this—a smart doctor listens to the nurses." That advice has stood me in good stead for the past 25 years as I practiced pediatrics.

My mother grew up on a small farm. Her dad farmed; her mom did sewing. All the children did odd jobs to help make ends meet. When she finished high school she went to work as an inspector in a nearby factory. She had a dream that she could save enough money to go to nursing school. After two years in the factory, she was almost ready. Then her little brother needed an operation, and there went all of her money, until an anonymous donor in her small town gave the needed money for nursing school. She never found out who it was but always suspected the town doctor.

She thrived in nursing school, and afterward she moved to a town that needed hospital nurses. In that hospital (in the closing days of World War II) she met my father, a handsome young sailor, sick with pneumonia, just mustered out of service.

When I was a kid, I was fascinated by her stories. I remember her excitement, telling me of the first blood transfusion she helped with, the first time she gave a dose of penicillin, of taking care of patients in iron lungs during the 1952 polio epidemic. I loved putting on her navy wool nurse's cape and pretending to wipe out disease.

When I was in high school, she was head nurse in the local ED. She looked so capable in her starched white uniform, lace-up Clinic shoes, and white nurse's cap with black velvet ribbon, I was sure she could handle anything.

She could diagnose at 40 paces, we all said. On weekends, I was allowed to come and watch. You never knew what would come through the door. When I was in college, and doing premed observations with local physicians, they would invariably suggest that I could learn more from watching my mom than anyone else. "She's seen it all," they said.

So when I went off to medical school (at the same school my mother attended), I was always conscious that I was walking the same halls she had trod 30 years earlier. When she came to visit, I showed off the new big city ED and she oohed and aahed at the equipment. In the NICU she beamed at tiny babies who wouldn't have survived when she was a student. When I didn't know what to do (such as what size umbilical artery catheter to ask for with my first 1,200-gram preemie), asking the nurse would put me on the right track. And when I spent my first week in practice as a pediatrician, I wished she were my office nurse, to help me with all of the real world issues I hadn't yet learned.

So here I am, after 10 years as an office pediatrician, four as a hospital administrator, and 12 as a pediatric hospitalist. Last night I took care of a patient with critical hypocalcemia, discovered only because an astute nurse noticed some subtle muscle twitching in the middle of the night. She was sure something wasn't right, even though the patient said he felt just fine. She called me, and I listened. A smart doctor listens to the nurses. ▼

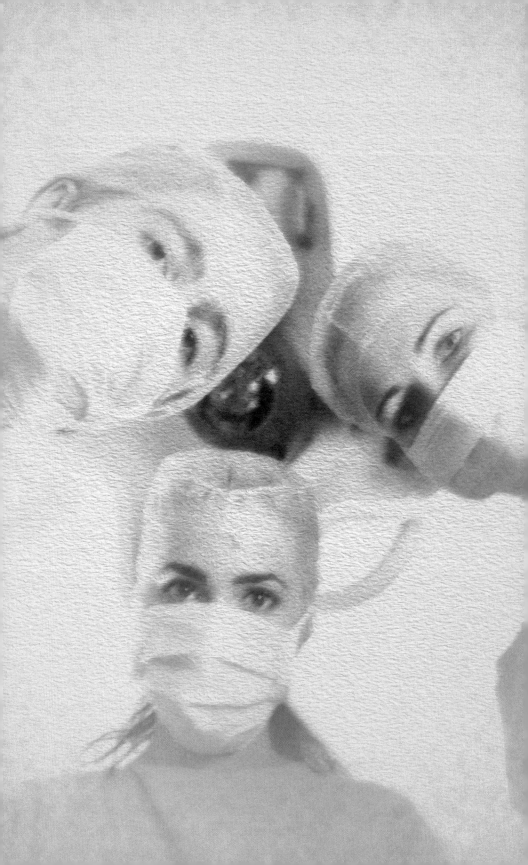

From the Other Side

Stories by patients or family members.

"I am grateful that our physician and nurses are repeatedly willing to set aside stoic professionalism and relate to me personally, letting me draw my cues from them, treating me like a friend who has been there for every up and down since the first diagnosis."

Amy Noel Green

Seized

A child's chronic illness may be impossible to control, but there's still a choice to make.

Jennifer K. Englund, MSEd

It begins with a gurgle from deep in Daney's throat: low, primal, guttural. In the next few seconds, her back will arch and her palms will turn up. Her 10-year-old self will twitch, then tremble, like she's being electrocuted—and in a way, she is.

Daney can't stop the seizures. I can't stop them. The only thing to do is to wait them out. To hope she does come out, to pray that if she does, she'll be the same girl who liked setting up her dollhouse, reading Nancy Drew books, and taking long walks.

After 116 seconds, the gurgles and trembling subside. My lap becomes wet from Daney's full surrender. Then, the worst part: Daney gasps laboriously for one breath. Her stomach draws in sharply and her ribs jut out. Back still arched, eyes still closed, my daughter lies in my arms—not moving, not breathing.

I wonder: Is this the last breath Daney will take? Is she in pain? Brain damaged? And I start crying because I can't do a single thing to fix any of this. I cry because I can't protect her, because I spoke unkindly to her earlier in the day when she struggled with her math homework. Because once or twice a month, I get this opportunity to evaluate and correct myself, and I still blow it.

Daney ... I try to say it gently, to hold back my urgency. I know she's already fighting with herself. She wants to come out of this; her body isn't letting her.

It's not fair this should happen to my girl. She's kind. She's bright. She plays plastic farm animals with her brothers. She bakes brownies, picks tulips, and sneaks love notes into her daddy's pockets.

This is how it will be, the neurologist has told me.

This is how it will be, my husband has said.

I've told myself I'll never get used to it. I haven't in three years and dozens of grand mal seizures.

In Daney's most terrible cluster of seizures, I held onto my daughter. While she lost herself, I got lost, too, in ED visits, CT scans, ambulance rides, EEGs. I didn't go to coffee with my friends. I didn't return phone calls. I moved Daney's bed into my room, and took her to work at the college with me. I gave up sleep, waiting vigilantly for the sign of a seizure, but also worrying at the silence. I ate little, and exercised less, and rarely played Legos with my boys. I was afraid for Daney, but also for myself. Would something happen where I'd have to take care of her forever? What would that mean to my future, to my fulfillment? If I lost her, how would I survive?

But after that terrible cluster, something happened: an ornery little bee stung the bottom of Daney's foot. And for three nights in a row, my girl was up, complaining and icing and hobbling around. She'd survived more than 20 violent seizures by that time. But this bump was making her crazy.

As I watched Daney stick her foot under the faucet at 2 AM, I suddenly realized that Daney had never whined, not once, about having epilepsy. Here was an adolescent girl who'd lain in a pool of drool and urine after a seizure, gone to the ED in nothing but frog panties. She'd missed school, couldn't go on all-day field trips or down the high slide or on sleepovers.

And I hadn't been able fix any of that. But Daney had never expected me to. Maybe my aching shoulders, constant headaches, and memory lapses were showing me that the neurologist and my husband had been right: that this was how it was going to be. That all I could do was to accept my daughter's epilepsy, to live with it—just like Daney did.

It's been three years now since the diagnosis, and Daney's seizures still come regularly; they will for a long time. Though I sometimes fight against accepting them as a normal part of my family's life, I've told myself that I can choose to worry, to wait, and to watch. Or I can know that I'm terrified, yes, and sad and incredibly sorry, but that that isn't going to make any of this better. I can choose to do yoga and have lunch with friends and engage my classes in lively discussions.

So now, as Daney lies in my lap, her chest finally falling then rising, I'm relieved—for her, for me. Her epilepsy and I may never be in complete harmony, but certain truths have gradually emerged: that although the seizures begin with a gurgle, there's no way to know how they'll end. That while Daney's disease has changed me, she has taught me how to live with it. That when the worry and the waiting and the seizures are stripped away, my daughter is right there—drawing faeries, making mud cakes, singing sweetly. ▼

The Brat

A patient remembers a nurse who hung in there.

Tiana Tozer

Jaime sets the tray on the bedside table and moves it in front of me.
I'm sullen. "No one else in ICU has to eat."

"No one else in ICU is conscious," she repies, with an indulgent smile
Lucky dogs.

Jaime, my nurse, has soft brown eyes in a kind face that's framed by
frizzy, dark brown, shoulder-length hair. Twenty days ago, completely
dependent on her, I hadn't even known her name as I took inventory of my
destroyed body.

"That doesn't look so good," I'd remarked, assessing my right-upper
bicep, black like a charred piece of driftwood.

"It's just bruised," she said. "It will heal."

"That's one hell of a bruise," I said, as if this were all normal for me.

"What's wrong with my legs?" I asked.

"They're broken," she said. She might have been speaking about the
weather. *Yes, today is sunny and very nice. Yes, your legs are broken.*

"Both of them?" I asked.

"Yes," she said.

Would you like fries with that?

Now, 20 days later, I can't imagine being here without her.

I only remember bits and pieces of the day or two after I was run over
by the car. Jaime fills in the blanks: "I waited with you in room 18 while
staff and equipment were gathered for your first trip to the OR."

"Was I conscious?" I ask.

"You were in and out," she says. "You asked me if you were in
heaven."

"What did you tell me?"

"I said 'no,' and thought to myself, if this is heaven, we're all in
trouble."

At her revelation, the right side of my mouth turns up. Almost a smile.

At 20 years old, life as I knew it has ended. My body has been irre-
vocably altered by severe leg injuries—to escape the pain, boredom, and
reality of my situation, I have regressed to the age of 10, possibly 14. In the
early days after my admission, the nurses would refer to me as "the leg,"
but by now I'm sure they're calling me "the brat." Because I am.

I plod through lunch, endure my second dressing change, and as I contemplate my limited choices to pass the time until dinner and the next dressing change, Jaime enters with a mischievous look on her face.

"Want to get out of this room?" she asks.

"Really?" My face brightens, then falls. "How?"

She gathers up the wires, tubes, and machines my body now requires and fastens it all to the bed. She drapes a large square sheet of plastic over my leg, throws open the glass doors of my room, and pushes my bed into the corridor. The wheels roll on the nondescript carpet. We pass through the giant gray double doors that lead out of the ICU and stop in the corridor just before the entrance to the OR. Sun shines through four bay windows.

Jaime moves my bed parallel to the windows. The view isn't much, just a fenced-off area cleared for a construction project: dirt and a chain-link fence. The mesh of the fence looks like a larger version of the skin grafts on my leg.

"That will be the new physicians and surgeons building," Jaime informs me. The sun streams through the glass and, like invisible ribbons, floats down onto my skin as if to provide me with the human contact I have been denied for the past weeks.

I watch people and cars move along the less than busy street. It's so colorful: red, blue, green, bathed in the yellow of the sun. I reach out and touch the warm glass. One of my blue machines erupts into shrill beeps. I ignore it. Jaime punches buttons and the shrieking stops. I take a deep breath and exhale.

There isn't much to look at, but it's enough. The corners of my mouth turn upward as I lie in front of the tall glass windows, basking in the sun's rays.

"Is that a smile?" Jaime teases.

"No." I give her a playful glare before I break into a grin.

For a moment, as I gaze out the window doing something normal, I am just a kid. It is a reprieve and a reminder of another world, a world I still think is within my reach.

It was Jaime who took me on bed walks to see the babies and cajoled me into an air bed to avoid pressure sores, Jaime whose boys drew me pictures, Jaime who was always patient, Jaime who I trusted and relied on.

Twenty-four years later, asking about her recollections for my memoir, I included a question I wasn't sure I wanted answered: "I was *so* awful. How did you get stuck with me?"

"I volunteered," she replied. "I liked you and wanted to help you recover. I also liked challenges, and your case from the standpoint of your wounds was challenging."

I smiled. She *chose* me. ▼

The Game of What If?

When he fought so hard to live, it seemed heartless to ask him how he wanted to die.

Susan Luton

My brother's partner Sean, my sister, and I had been spending more time together than usual—keeping vigil over my heavily sedated brother, who was lying in an ICU room in Los Angeles. He'd fallen and split his head open—I'd assumed it was because his legs were weakened by the drugs he took to battle a brain tumor (Tommy Tumor, my brother called it), but the doctors said a clot had broken loose inside Ryan's leg and butterflied into his lungs, causing him to lose consciousness.

His left arm and leg had stopped moving, probably because of the impact of the fall on the tumor. Then a superbug made its appearance, and a killer antibiotic started flowing through one of his many tubes. Even if Ryan recovered, he might spend the rest of his life in bed, connected to a ventilator.

Not a sound had left my brother since his fall. We three "vigilants"— as I'd taken to calling us—took turns at his side, talking soothingly and touching him, wanting to believe the nurse who said this might help restore him to consciousness. Every once in a while he would lightly squeeze someone's hand. When a doctor told us that it was simply a reflex, we paid no attention.

Then one night my brother jerked his breathing tube halfway out of his throat while an X-ray technician had her head turned away. Everyone assured us that Ryan's action wasn't premeditated; that his level of consciousness was only foglike; that he couldn't have seen the tech's turned head, since a nurse had recently lubricated his eyes, which hadn't been fully closed for days, and put patches on them.

When I got there the next day and saw the restraints pinning down my brother's hands, I knew that the chances he'd ever talk to us were even more minuscule. And I desperately wanted him to talk—if only for long enough to tell us what he'd decided should be the maximum number of tubes going in and out of him. Or how many times he wanted the doctors to test whether he could breathe on his own, note his agitation when he couldn't, and then up the sedative dose. Maybe he'd tell us, "You've been here all this time? Humph. *I* was in a tertiary universe. Quite pleasant."

Or maybe he'd turn an accusing eye on us and scold, "Why haven't you picked up my signal that I'm ready to go? I even tried pulling out that oxygen-breathing snake that's been clogging my throat."

This last *may be* gave me pause. My brother had spent the past year making enormous physical and emotional concessions. He'd done it with an almost regal dignity. But I felt a deep doubt about the dignity of his present situation—just that morning, an additional monitoring machine, two additional tubes filled with secretions.

When I shared this doubt with my brother's physician, he said that Ryan probably wasn't ready to give up yet. Then he launched into a jargon-filled account of my brother's many complications over the past year. "But it's a philosophical question," I countered. "How willing are doctors to say, 'There's no more point to this'?" He assured me that, for them, "pointless is pointless," and that, yes, in a few days or weeks he and the other doctors might be asking us vigilants, "Do we attempt another course of treatment? Or stop treatment altogether?"

Later I turned to Sean for clues: "Did you and Ryan ever talk about if and when to bring everything to a halt?" Sean said that the only usable information, despite all their long conversations, despite the health care proxy form, was that Ryan didn't want to continue living if his mind were gone. "How can anyone cover *all* the bases?" Sean asked. "Besides, Ryan didn't want to talk about such things."

It was true. Almost until his fall, my brother was still insisting that he'd beat Tommy Tumor. None of us had been strong enough or—as it seemed at the time—heartless enough to play "what if?" with Ryan, to make him envision his dying.

Ryan's condition continued to deteriorate.

One night I dreamt that I was working at a crowded festival. My job was to take lunch plates to the festival-goers who had ordered them. I jostled my way through bodies for a long time, struggling to keep the food from sliding off the plates. When I finally found the right people and delivered the food, my brother appeared. "Why did you take that winding route?" he asked me. "Look over there." He pointed to the food preparation area. It was a short, direct distance from where we stood.

The next morning I told Sean and my sister that it was time to stop life support. They agreed. My brother died a few days later. ▼

The Third Way

ECT isn't what it used to be.

Andrew Merton

On January 2, 2007, 11 AM, at McLean Hospital in Belmont, Massachusetts, I lay on a gurney, fully clothed, awaiting the first of seven rounds of electroconvulsive therapy—aka ECT, aka "shock therapy." An anesthetist named Anne Marie said, "You'll feel a pinch," and slid a needle into my right arm. Moments later I felt the delirious rush of oncoming oblivion, followed by blessed nothingness.

I am 64, married, with two grown children. I teach. I write. I enjoy life with my family. Except when I am in a depression.

Depression is painful, debilitating, pervasive, and enduring. That is why, when I am depressed, I flirt with Ms. Death the way some men flirt with younger women. She flirts back, a temptress in basic black.

One night in 1974 I gave in, swallowing half a bottle of sleeping pills. I awoke 36 hours later, relieved but also disappointed.

In May 2006 I ended my most recent round of talk therapy, which had been helpful, and weaned myself from the antidepressant Effexor, which, while curbing my depression, had also induced chronic drowsiness, a craving for alcohol, and a sometimes antisocial attitude. Over the years I have tried many other medications, alone or in combination. None provided the relief I sought. Now I was determined to do without. I continued to see my psychiatrist for the month it took to quit Effexor. The withdrawal went smoothly.

But in September I tumbled into a severe depression. I taught badly. I wrote nothing. Ordinary conversation became painfully difficult, so I avoided people. Ms. D hovered, wearing something slinky, off-the-shoulder. What are you waiting for? she whispered.

In October I happened across an excerpt from *Shock: The Healing Power of Electroconvulsive Therapy*, by Kitty Dukakis and Larry Tye. Dukakis credited ECT with saving her life. Tye contributed a thorough history of ECT, from its initial use as a treatment for epilepsy, to its misuse as an agent of control and punishment in public psychiatric hospitals in the '50s and '60s (dramatized in *One Flew Over the Cuckoo's Nest*, in which the character played by Jack Nicholson endures an ECT-induced seizure with no anesthesia), to its refinement into a frequently effective treatment for unresponsive depression and severe mood swings.

I thought, why not? I was scheduled for a second semester sabbatical. I called the ECT unit at McLean and made an appointment for an evaluation, an all-day affair that included a physical exam, a blood workup, and a 90-minute consultation with a psychiatrist. He warned me that ECT usually resulted in a period of short-term memory loss and that, as with any procedure involving general anesthesia, there was a slight risk of death. I thought, but did not say, only *slight?*

January 2, 11:30 AM: I awoke in a recovery room. A cheerful nurse named Cecelia asked me how I was doing. "Fine," I said, by which I meant that I was in no pain but too hazy to articulate the fact. After about an hour, which included a brief interview with Dr. Seiner, the psychiatrist who had administered the treatment, I left the hospital with the friend who had driven me there that morning. The only physical indication that anything had happened to my head was a residue of gel on the right side.

Each of my six subsequent visits, spaced out over the next 16 days, was essentially the same. Later Dr. Seiner filled me in:

The ingredients in Anne Marie's potent cocktail were methohexital, a short-acting barbiturate anesthetic, and succinylcholine, a muscle relaxant, followed by propofol, after the treatment, to prolong sleep and promote a comfortable awakening.

The unilateral shock (up to 576 millicoulombs of charge, in some cases) was administered on the right side of my head and lasted from two to six seconds. (During bilateral ECT, by contrast, both sides of the brain are shocked, but with considerably less energy.) The duration of the seizure induced by the shock was typically one to two minutes. I was unconscious for about 10 minutes and more fully awake after 20 to 25 minutes.

During the immediate aftershock, Cecelia and the other nurses were patient and compassionate, open to conversations about work, family, movies, the weather. They provided invaluable—how else to put this?—grounding.

When I walked out of the hospital after my final treatment, I was dazed and without ambition. My short-term memory seemed to have eloped with my attention span and run off to Bali. For the next three months I did nothing that required much thought or volition.

But if I was inert, I was also content. Music, mostly Bach, helped. The lady in black, having no interest in contentment, slipped away unnoticed. My short-term memory returned gradually, along with my desire to work, and to play. This year, my wife and I celebrated our 30th anniversary, touring the Canadian Maritimes. And while small wisps of depression will always pester me, the big one, so far, has not returned. ▼

Every Three Months

A mother finds comfort in the emotional engagement of her son's nurses and physicians.

Amy Noel Green

I have had the unsettling experience of being told, on three different occasions, that my son's death was imminent. I know the routine now. Every three months we get an MRI, and if the news is good, every nurse who passes us will smile, or even mention in the waiting room that "the scans look real good." When the news is good, no one minds ruining the surprise.

The bad news is different. We are left sitting alone, and nurses who pass by either don't make eye contact or make uncomfortable small talk, avoiding the topic so obviously that what they aren't saying speaks volumes.

When the news is especially bad, the room we are taken to has a team waiting in it, fully assembled, each waiting to share their piece of information about the new reality we're facing.

My son Joel has been battling an atypical teratoid/rhabdoid (AT/RT) brain tumor for three years. He was diagnosed at age one, and his first recurrence was in October, three months before his second birthday. He was given a few weeks to maybe four months to live, and we were told that although it was likely he'd be alive at Christmas, he probably wouldn't be comfortable.

"This is a tragedy," our neuro-oncologist told us, with tears in his eyes. Our two favorite nurses—the ones who had made the long days in the infusion room almost bearable because of their willingness to laugh with me—were already crying. The shared love of this team released our own tears, previously bottled up by shock.

We are people of faith, and we believe a series of miracles led to Joel's five-month remission on palliative care. The tumors that eventually returned came one at a time, instead of exploding all over his brain as predicted. Some nurses shared our faith, and some did not, but all were willing to answer our practical questions about science, medical expectations, and our son's continued care without belittling our beliefs. Whether they thought Joel was "a miracle baby" or just one of the beautiful, unexplainable exceptions, their joy—when it became obvious that Joel was living and not dying—is something I will never forget.

Last year, 11 months after Joel was declared terminal, we were escorted into a room with our neuro-oncologist, two nurses, and an oncology social worker (the social worker was a giveaway that the news would be devastating). "Joel has three new tumors," we were told, "two in his brain and one in his spine. We don't know how to explain the year you've had, but this is what we were expecting a year ago when we told you he was dying." How were we all together again, a year later, crying in an exam room, reliving the worst moment of my life?

Amazingly, two months later, Joel's MRI showed that the two tumors in his brain were gone: they had resolved on just palliative treatment. The tumor in his spine was shrinking. Our neuro-oncologist had eager company, our nurses, as he came to deliver the news, and there was shocked joking as we rejoiced that Joel was, once again, defying the odds.

This last year has been incredible. After cheating death twice, our son was beginning to catch up. He could swallow solid foods again and had finally begun to walk. We even had five amazing months with no treatment whatsoever, not even palliative at-home chemotherapy. After so many good MRIs that we thought we were finally in the clear, just over 12 months from the last declaration that Joel would not live much longer (and a few months before his fourth birthday), Joel had another bad MRI. It showed a large tumor in his spine, growing much more quickly than all the other recurrences.

"I believe this level of growth represents a new phase in his disease," said his physician, adding that Joel would not see more remissions of the sort he'd had in the past but was "entering the downward spiral."

How does our team continue to deliver this roller coaster of news? They live it with us, happy when we are happy, sad when we are sad. They are very clear with us about what to expect, and yet they hold a little of our hope. There is no easy way to hear, three times, that your son is about to die. But given a choice, I would always rather hear it from someone who expresses love for my son. I am grateful that our physician and nurses are repeatedly willing to set aside stoic professionalism and relate to me personally, letting me draw my cues from them, treating me like a friend who has been there for every up and down since the first diagnosis. ▼

Intake Interview

Gender: it's not an emergency, is it?

Joy Ladin

The chest pains—short, sharp, and frequent—had started in the early afternoon. I had been painting my children's faces and pulling a picnic together at the home of my wife; we're separated. When she appeared in the kitchen, I went home, shaved, changed into a skirt and blouse, rushed on some lipstick and foundation, and drove myself to the hospital.

Our local hospital is small and familial. All three of our children were born there. It was an early summer evening and business was slow, so as a woman with chest pains I got a lot of attention.

"Next of kin?" the intake clerk asked me. "Husband?" she asked, smiling, when I gave her the name. "Wife," I replied (my wife's name is gender neutral). I was grateful that marital laws in Massachusetts enabled me to pass as a married lesbian. "Oh, that's fine," she said, her tone carefully neutral, and handed me off to the ED intake nurse.

"Are you still having periods?" she asked. "No," I said. It was the truth, more or less.

They gave me a room and a gown right away. No one likes hospital gowns, but for someone with a female chest and male genitalia, they hold a particular horror. I decided to leave my skirt on.

A nurse wheeled in the electrocardiograph. We joked as she placed cold adhesive sensors all over my chest. "I don't have to expose anything," she said, as her hands moved toward my breasts. Unfortunately, she did. "I have to ask you some really bizarre questions now," she told me. The first was about ethnicity. "The state requires it," she said apologetically. She glanced down at the next question on her list.

"Are you physically male or female?" I hesitated. This was the first time anyone had questioned my gender, at least to my face. I wondered how I'd given myself away. I'd put on my lipstick correctly, the hair on my head was long enough, and the hair on my face was sparse enough. My voice was strained, but I'd hoped they would attribute that to stress rather than to my do-it-yourself voice training.

"Physically male. Unfortunately," I said. "I'm trans."

Hoping I sounded curious rather than humiliated, I added, "Why did you ask?" The American Medical Association, after years of reports of transgender patients dying because physicians refused to treat them, had passed guidelines stating that treating people like me is a professional obligation. But transphobia is more deeply ingrained in our culture than homophobia, and I had no desire to encounter it when I might be dying.

"Oh, they make us ask everyone that question," she answered. "We're trying to get these questions changed. The only one that's relevant is ethnicity." She was wrong. Gender, I was discovering, is relevant to every aspect of emergency health care.

She left me alone, and about a half hour later another nurse arrived. I wondered how much she knew about me.

"Do you shave your arms?" she asked. And suddenly I saw what she saw: patches of the short black hair that seems to spring up the moment I stop running the razor over my skin. Testosterone-inspired body hair is different from estrogenized body hair; it's darker and coarser, and it grows every which way. "Yes," I answered at last, my strained voice shredding. Real women don't shave their arms.

"Are your feet cold?" she asked. I hadn't realized it, but they were. She slid a pair of thick, beige socks across to me.

She was smiling. Why was she smiling? "Heart attacks," she said, "present differently in women than in men. The symptoms are vaguer, and *we*"—she emphasized the word slightly—"are much more likely to ignore them." She laughed. "We're just stronger than they are." I tried to match her conspiratorial smile.

"You have to ignore pain to take care of kids," I said. It was the truth, but it felt like a lie.

"That's for sure," she agreed.

"I waited as long as I could," I said, wanting some kind of affirmation—or was it absolution?—from her. "The pain kept getting worse," I croaked, "and I finally decided—" I broke off.

"Of course you needed to come in," she said. "Someone's taking care of the kids, right?"

"Yes," I said thickly.

"Well, then you have to take care of yourself." I couldn't speak anymore. I just nodded.

"Does it hurt to talk?" Very little was left of the voice I'd worked so hard to develop.

"No," I said, although it did. "This is the way I always sound when I'm upset." ▼

A Passing Shadow

The 'what ifs' can multiply when a loved one survives cancer.

Gail Lukasik, MA, PhD

My husband and I wake into the narrow December dark. He brushes his teeth, dresses, then busies himself as I eat breakfast. His packed suitcase sits by the back door. It's 5 AM, two days before Thanksgiving. At precisely 9 AM, the surgeon will remove my husband's right kidney, the one he is 99% sure is cancerous.

The house has a quiet ticking sound—the furnace clicks on, the clock's minute hand slowly advances. We don't say what we are both thinking—how he could die. Instead, we talk about other things. How I'll come home after the surgery and see to the dog, how fortunate it is that the hospital is five minutes from our house, how (barring no heavy city traffic) our daughter should arrive around nine, how our son will fly into O'Hare next week—plans predicated on our conviction, based on nothing but our need to believe it, that everything will be all right.

And while we're talking, I'm trying not to see how glazed his blue eyes are with fear.

I tell him once again my belief that this isn't cancer, that until it's confirmed, I'm clinging to the 1% chance. A kind of magical thinking I've fallen into since this all began allows me to function, because I've yet to take it all in.

Just two weeks ago, my husband stood in the family room and told me he had cancer. And though I was hearing and understanding him, I refused to believe what he said. For a moment I even considered that he might be joking.

We stood there for what seemed like forever, until I finally heard him, until I understood that the slight pain in his back we'd thought was his gall bladder wasn't.

After that, for the two weeks before the surgery, we soothed ourselves with "what ifs"—a way to defer the inevitable "why me?"

What if the technician who performed the MRI on his gall bladder *hadn't* moved the scan beyond the required area? Was she following a hunch, or was she just being thorough? What if that day she'd been tired or distracted? What if she hadn't seen the dark shadow?

Then right now we'd be asleep, warm in our bed, living without fear. No one would be cut open today. And cancer might be growing quietly, but surely, inside him.

The surgery takes too long. My daughter and I sit through the morning as the other family members are called. We reassure each other that this is a big surgery. But after two hours have passed, the two hours predicted by the surgeon for the operation, we begin to worry in earnest. I ask the waiting room volunteer what she knows. She says, "He's still in surgery."

Finally, the surgeon and his assistant come into the waiting room and tell us the surgery went well and that the cancer was encapsulated within the kidney. Which means he doesn't need chemotherapy or radiation?

"It was a surgical cure," the surgeon explains.

"A surgical cure?" I ask, as if he's speaking a foreign language, still not wanting to accept that it was cancer.

"The surgery *was* the cure," he smiles wearily. "It was the best outcome we could hope for."

It's too much to take in; my mind shuts down. My daughter has to repeat the surgeon's instructions of where we should wait for my husband to be wheeled out of the recovery room.

While we wait by the surgery doors, they wheel out a man who's just had gall bladder surgery. He looks as bad as anyone can and still be alive. I am faint with apprehension. My daughter tells me to sit down. When they wheel out my husband, he's joking with the nurses, who are laughing and joking along with him. The smiles on the nurses' faces and their lighthearted mood lift the somberness of the moment. My husband looks so good to me.

Those next few days we cling to whatever humor we can find. On day two of his recovery, my husband wakes from his morphine sleep and points to a plant that has just been delivered to his room.

"Who's that from?" he asks.

"Your sister, Kathy," I tell him.

"Oh," he says, and goes back to sleep. And when he wakes hours later, he points to the plant again.

"Who's that from?"

My daughter and I exchange glances and smiles.

"Dad," she says, "it's from Aunt Kathy."

And he falls back to sleep.

Thanksgiving Day, my daughter and I sit in his room, while he dozes and wakes and we watch football games and nibble on the Thanksgiving dinner that he barely eats. And I think, *it's going to be okay*. He's going to be okay. It is enough for now. And I'm so very thankful. ▼

A Stone of Contention

Competence and bedside manner don't always go hand in hand.

Tim Bascom

At the hospital, when the emergency medical technician (EMT) eases me into a lying position on the gurney, I curl up, clenching like a possum around the spiked ball of pain in my right flank.

"You need to breathe," says the EMT.

Cathy says, "He had kidney stones once. Could that be the problem?"

Breathe in through the nose, I think. Now out through the mouth. Or is it the other way? My hazy memories of Lamaze are no help.

The EMT looms back into view. "We called urology. They said Dr. Mercer is available."

Cathy and I stare at each other in distress. The EMT adds, "Not your top choice, eh? I tell you what, I'll check with the office once more."

I am already panicking. After going to Dr. Mercer for a vasectomy, I found myself walking bowlegged. I had developed an infected prostate accompanied by a burning bladder and aching testicles. After two months of antibiotics, I was still subject to painful relapses, yet Dr. Mercer was as comforting as a rodeo clown.

"I can barely walk," I explained to him.

"Just think, no more babies," he shot back.

"But I mean I hurt down there all the time."

"Heck of a thing, eh. Can't live with 'em, can't live without 'em."

Suing was not my style. However, I had written him a good-riddance letter, making it clear that I not only found his remarks inappropriate, I also suspected him of incompetence.

The EMT leans over me, shaking his head. "I'm afraid you're out of luck, buddy. It's either Mercer or another hospital."

"Look," he adds, "for what it's worth, I've worked with the guy. I know how difficult he is. But if he has to operate, he's good."

Cathy looks at me with worried eyes.

"Alright," I find myself whispering.

When the EMT comes back, he is chuckling: "You should have heard Mercer. He kept asking 'Are you *sure* we're talking about the same guy?'"

For the next hour I lie on a frigid X-ray table, being turned onto my cramped sides. The pain eases, and I wonder if a kidney stone has worked itself loose or if the Demerol has finally kicked in. Then Dr. Mercer strolls in, working a wad of gum and lifting dark aviator glasses to his forehead.

"Howdy pardner. How you doin'?"

"I've had better days," I say.

He nods. "I can see why. You've got a stone in there the size of a watermelon seed."

"Is it moving? Because the pain's improved."

He shakes his head. "You're leaking."

"Leaking?"

"It's like anything with pressure. Something has to give. In your case, the ureter popped. No pressure, no pain. You're fine for now, but after 24 hours, you're gonna be miserable. The bowels will shut down. A hundred years ago, I don't know...."

I try to assimilate this not-so-subtle hint. "So what do you recommend?"

"Well, if I was your brother, I'd say let's scope it and take that stone out."

I study his face closely. "And if you *were* my brother," I reply, "I guess I'd tell you to go ahead."

Did I just say that? What if he screws up? What if, subconsciously, he *wants* to screw up?

"I know we've had our differences," I add, "but I hope we can put that behind us."

"No problem, pardner." He stops at the door, lowering his sunglasses onto the bridge of his nose. "But I want you to know I'm good at this scoping stuff. Damn good."

As they strap my legs apart, I am ready to go under. The anesthesiologist says he is starting the anesthesia. I wonder why I am still alert enough to respond.

Suddenly, though, I'm staring up at a bowl of bright white light, and my throat feels like someone put a blow-dryer down it. I cough.

"Breathe through nose," says a disembodied woman.

"Have they started?" I croak.

"All over," says the woman. "So happy for you. Stone gone."

This voice is oddly familiar. The thin brows, too, when she leans in closer, pushing back black bangs.

"God is so good, don't you think?" she says. She begins to sing softly: "God is so good. God is so good."

Then it comes to me. This is the same recovery nurse who brought our son out of anesthesia when he had ear tube surgery. This is the woman who jostled him in her arms like she was mixing pancake batter in a Tupperware container, who insisted "baby need stimulus," dancing away from me as Luke reached and screamed. I had to pry him out of her hands;

he was so traumatized that, months later, he howled when he heard some-one with a similar accent.

Helplessness is a strange thing, I think, as this nurse putters around me, checking my IV and humming. Would I have ever turned to these two people if not forced?

She begins to sing again—"God is so good." I know that song from junior high. It is the sort of sentimental campfire tune that makes me roll my eyes, but now it seems strangely right. I feel so good lying here—set free from the tearing pain and the old resentments—that I could almost sing along. If it weren't for my dried-out throat, I would. ▼

Swabbing Tubby

Family caregiving can be trying on many levels, but a little levity may help.

Susan Clements

In retrospect, I can't help feeling sorry for the earnest young woman who tried so hard to show my mother, my sister, and myself how to hook up our brand-new, at-home, IV feeding device. She was all of 25, with the freshly scrubbed look of a young schoolgirl. Her youthful perkiness was no match for the trio of exhausted, crabby women who faced her across the empty hospital bed. Dad was down in X-ray having yet another CT scan, and the three of us were awaiting instructions on do-it-yourself intravenous feeding.

After the last surgery, my father had about a third of a functioning intestine. In order for him to absorb enough nutrition to survive, his surgeon prescribed liquid protein pumped directly into his veins via a central line implanted in his shoulder. The elusive Dr. Robertson, who could never be found when we wanted to ask him a question, left orders for us to hook Dad up to the IV pump at bedtime and unhook him in the morning.

My mother could never get the hang of programming the VCR, so the prospect of her operating this high-tech pump seemed a little daunting. But stoicism runs in the family, and we prepared to learn what we had to do to keep Dad alive.

"This looks complicated, Mrs. C, but we're going to take it one step at a time," said Sandra, our IV tutor. "Okay?"

"Okay," we three chorused, grimly facing the challenge.

The lesson was going smoothly as she pointed out all the knobs, dials, and indicators on the portable IV pump that would be delivered to our house later that week. We were all in a hospital-induced fugue state, so we continued to nod, pretending that we knew what she was talking about.

"It is very important that the needle and port stay sterile," Sandra said slowly, as if speaking to third graders. "We don't want any infections to happen, okay?"

"Okay." My mother looked like an especially formidable Buddha as she examined the tubes and needles encased in plastic.

"Now, you must wipe the port with this Betadine swab before inserting the needle. We're going to practice on this, okay?" Her voice bounced up at the end of every sentence.

The bed was covered with an array of plastic tubing, disposable needles, swabs, and latex gloves. Sandra reached into her tote and pulled out a plastic Country Crock margarine container with a rubber IV port implanted in its lid.

A wave of panicked hilarity arose in me. "Here's your swab... do you want to try it too?" said Sandra. We obediently opened our Betadine swabs. Mom went first, making two tentative swipes.

"Very good, Mrs. C!"

I followed, and passed the tub to my sister, like a pistol in Russian roulette.

"Okay, that was great!" said Sandra. "Do you have any questions?" We shook our heads in mute unison.

"Let's just review this one more time, okay?"

"Okay."

She asked us to show her that we remembered what to do, so the three of us went through the motions of hooking up the bag, adjusting the settings on the pump, and attaching the needle to the plastic tubing, being careful to keep everything sterile. We were proving to be model students, until we got to the margarine container representing my father's left shoulder.

"Time to swab tubby," said my sister.

"Yes, time to swab tubby!" I chimed in.

Sandra looked to my mother for the necessary gravitas.

"Now I'm swabbing tubby," said Mom.

"Okay, I see you've got it." She looked from Mom, to me, to my sister, then threw her arms out wide in a posture of benediction. "Feelings?"

I willed my face into a frozen mask. Mom and my sister were similarly Botoxed. We shook our heads vigorously.

Sandra hastily packed up her tote with all the plastic and tubes and left us with her card and some pamphlets, urging us to call her if we had any questions.

That pump never worked right. We woke to its insistent alarm almost every night, and in the end, it didn't lengthen my father's life more than a month or two. It wasn't Sandra's fault. She did her best to show us what we needed to do. It wasn't our fault either, or even the elusive Dr. Robertson's. Dad eventually succumbed to one last infection, even though every day we faithfully swabbed tubby. ▼

To the Child They Were All One Kind

Most gave comfort; one brought her the moon.

Sandra Stone

I called them all "Nurse" for a long time before I came to distinguish those who brought meds from those who tended, those who manipulated my joints from those who tried to interest me in pegs and rods. Then, too, there were those who got in the pool with me and tried to get my knees to bend, those two afflicted stems with bulbous centers.

I treasure a small, fan-folded book I keep on my nightstand. I can see only page by page. In this way time is stilled. I squint at the faded images, at my notations in pencil. There's the autograph I still have from Woodsy, a tall blonde with mischievous blue eyes—Woodsy, an occupational therapist who specialized in the orthopedic care of children. "Yours, under the moon and those stars."

You would not believe what Woodsy pulled off, despite the strict rules of the hospital administration. Today socialization and mental well-being are crucial parts of any care plan, especially for children. In 1948 they were unheard of.

I was still nonambulatory after two years of hospitalization with what was at first believed to be traumatic-onset juvenile rheumatoid arthritis. On the afternoon before I was to be discharged to a rehabilitation facility—a pretend child, watchful and joyless among dying and broken children—Woodsy said to me, as I finished lacing a leather wallet, a craft project I hated, "I'm taking you on an adventure tonight. Dress up. Don't forget to pack your toothbrush."

"What?" I exclaimed. "Where could we be going? And who says so?"

"I've taken care of all that," Woodsy said. Her eyes crinkled when she smiled.

"I don't know you that well," I grumbled.

True, I had had occupational therapy once a week. But I made strenuous objection to its purpose—to amuse me. I was not amused. I preferred to be a bookworm. Woodsy do-si-doed around my wheelchair; she was that pleased. "Be ready at five," she said, braking me at the entrance to my ward.

Oh, the fuss that was made over me that night, how my hair was done up by one of the aides, how clothes (real clothes, that must have been stored for me at the time of my admission) were now brought out. Glass beads. I hadn't seen myself in a mirror in two years. I knew the word *puberty*, but not what transformations it brought about.

Woodsy wheeled me into the elevator, the same one that, clanking, brought the washing machines up to boil the towels. (It was the year of the great polio epidemic.) My diagnosis had grown fuzzier. I was a conundrum to the physicians, an odd duck, the most ambulatory of the nonambulant. Why should I tell them the secret of my swollen knees: no one knew daddy had just died. *Put the past in your lock box. Look to the future*, was what the grown-ups had said. This was before the enlightenment of grief therapy.

"Where are we going?" I demanded. When the doors opened, I was unprepared. There, spread before me, was the tarpaper roof of the hospital, obstructed by duct work, heating equipment, chimneys, with no guardrail, and a view of the great hazy chasm that was the City of Angels. Before I could open my mouth, Woodsy maneuvered me into a position where I could see at once what was in store for me. Two metal beds with sleeping bags, side by side. One chair and a card table with a checkered cloth set out. A potted geranium for a centerpiece.

There was a picnic basket that had been wrapped gaily by the kitchen. Best of all, from Woodsy, a gold foil–jacketed edition of Walt Whitman's *Leaves of Grass*. I kept the foil for years, the book forever, and with it, the image of Woodsy. Could she have been past 22?

What arguments must have gone on behind closed doors for Woodsy to arrange this splendor for her most irritable patient?

Woodsy, wherever you are, that was my first epiphany. I soared through stars. I felt myself standing, walking to a less hazarded place. And the possibility of being, if not beautiful, wise.

Sky was a dense navy blue tarp. Pinpricks of light exceeded their competence. Woodsy and I, separate bundles, lay summers apart, campfires, river runs, sunlit glades between us. Woodsy was the best overnighter ever. She told me if I had one moon, I had a guardian friend. She read aloud to me from Whitman, "Song of the Open Road."

For all the clinicians who came after, for those who would remember the ideals with which they set out in their profession, I pass down the legend of Woodsy, who made a starstruck 13-year-old less a child of the *limberlost*. For who among us does not need a personal moon, a sky raining stars, and a trail that leads to the open road? ▼

Breathing Room

Did she invite this illness?

Linda Meierhoffer, MS, MPA, BA

A s we pulled into the hotel parking lot in Gallup, New Mexico, I flipped open my blinking cell phone and saw two voice mails and a text message from my gynecologist. When I reached her later that evening she said she'd consulted with an oncologist about the lesion she'd noticed during my recent dilation and curettage; because of previous biopsy results and abnormal Pap smears, I was at risk for cancer and needed a complete hysterectomy.

The timing was lousy: my husband Mark and I were driving from Kansas City to Palm Springs, California, for three months in a rented house, where we planned to work surrounded by the crimson bougainvillea and desert sun we loved. Though my doctor recommended that we come right back, we decided to push on to Palm Springs and stay there for the rest of January.

Far too soon, I was back home in February's deep freeze, on my way into a bright and shiny operating room. Although the operation went smoothly and my postoperative pathology results showed that the lesion was benign, three weeks later a large clot threatened to burst my freshly stapled abdominal incision.

I felt like my tidy life was coming unwound. Instead of salvaging some last bit of our long-awaited winter escape, I'd be operated on again. I was 51, exactly the age my father had been the last time I saw him alive, as he was wheeled into an OR for cancer surgery. And my mother had been just 50 when she'd died of a cerebral hemorrhage. As I let go of Mark's hand and watched my daughter Megan's face, the nurses wheeled me through the OR doors, and I wondered if I would ever see my family again.

Afterwards, all the beds were full on the surgical unit, so I was transferred from the recovery room to the oncology floor. Four North was filled with bald-headed, battle-scarred patients. Depressed that I was once again tethered to a catheter bag and iv pole, afraid that the clot would return, and angry that I couldn't control what was happening to me, I counted the minutes until my next push of morphine and the number of steps it took for me to creep, bent at the waist, to the bathroom. I was in a dark place that I had never known existed, one where a lack of hormones and sleep were infused with fear and the remnants of anesthesia.

"Do you ever think of harming yourself?" my doctor asked, as I sat slumped against the lumpy pillows, my expression flat, tears slipping down my chin and onto my neck. "No," I said, "but for the first time I can understand what makes someone want to."

Had I invited this surgery? Had I tempted death with the unspoken fear that I'd die young like Mama and Daddy? I thought of my first yoga teacher, whose behavior was sometimes as unbalanced as I was as a new student in tree pose, and what she'd told us once in class: "People open themselves up to disease and let it in." While some small part of me wanted to get better, go back to California with Mark, and be around to watch our kids get married and have children, I cried more during those four days in the hospital than I'd cried in 40 years.

The night before I was released, I dreamed I was under water. I awoke gasping, with panic that coursed from my abdomen to my throat. I grabbed for the call button. Jeff, the night-shift RN, was there in moments. "Help me," I whispered. "I'm drowning."

In a soothing voice, he talked until the anxiety released itself from my chest, my arms, my wide-open eyes. He fed me ice chips, straightened my twisted blankets, and gave me a pill to help me sleep; his gentle touch was something I had not had since I was a scared little girl and my mother stroked my head when the lightning danced on my bedroom walls at night.

In the morning, Jeff brought his little girl to meet me and see the picture of my cat I'd placed on the windowsill to keep me company. Her stepmother was a nurse at the same hospital; her shift began just as Jeff's ended, and she'd bring Jeff's daughter to work so that Jeff could drive her home.

That afternoon before I was discharged, my own daughter Megan came from work dressed in a pinstriped suit. I started to cry when I saw her, all grown up and about the same age I was when she was born. "Don't, Mom, you'll make me start," she told me.

I had crazy clown hair, roughed up and sticking out from all the tossing I'd done the night before. "Wow, you don't look so good," she said with a laugh as she sat down next to me. Without another word, Megan picked up the comb from my bedside table and began to smooth my hair.

Only weeks later did I learn that Jeff's first wife had died of cancer several years earlier, leaving his little girl without a mother. I figure he knew exactly how it felt to hope for breath and wonder where the air would come from. ▼

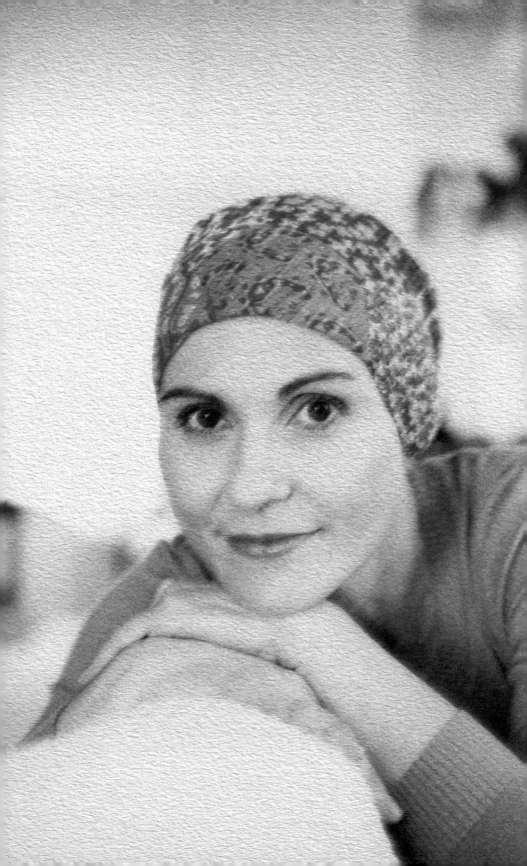

Tables Turned

When the nurse becomes the patient.

"Although I'd been a nurse for more than 20 years, this was the first time I had been so completely dependent on the health care system. I felt vulnerable. I knew too much."

Alice C. Facente, MSN, RN-BC

To Mania and Back

Becoming more than a number on a wristband.

Joan Schmidt, MS–MPH, RN, ACRN

It all started after a colleague jumped to her death from a 15th-floor balcony. Rumors spread that she leapt in uniform, clutching her agency-issued pen-based computer and paperwork. But questions posed by the staff about the incident were dismissed by the leaders of the home agency as "morbid curiosity."

I was an HIV–AIDS specialist with a dual master's degree; for 23 years my career flourished. But I became increasingly troubled by the silence surrounding my colleague's death, and for three days I called around looking for answers. My anxiety escalated. Soon, painful memories came flooding back.

My mother, a World War II Army nurse, first attempted suicide one month after my 11th birthday. It was Thanksgiving week; she slashed her throat with a razor blade. From that day on she veered between the vibrant, nurturing mother she had once been and a paranoid "crazy lady" who conversed with God, angels, and saints in our dish cabinets. Eventually, she left the house only to go to church, spending most of her time wandering like specter, a haunted look in her eyes. Psychiatrists have since told me that she must have been either paranoid schizophrenic or schizo-affective—either way, psychiatry in the 1950s and 1960s couldn't restore her mental health. When she died in 1985 of liver cirrhosis and addiction to barbiturates, narcotics, and sedatives, I'd lied to friends and associates. Fearful of exposing a family history of mental disease, I told them she'd died of a stroke.

Within days of my colleague's suicide, I began telling colleagues, friends, and loved ones about my mother's illness and my fears that "vampire mommy" would rise from the grave to harm my family. I talked about her for three days straight and slept just two hours a night. I became hoarse from talking so much.

My husband listened quietly at first, then became increasingly alarmed. I wouldn't stop talking and I couldn't sleep—a deprivation that was impairing my judgment. My friends also listened patiently, but when the Neurontin my therapist prescribed failed to stop the escalating mania, two of my friends—one a nurse, the other a psychiatric social worker—convinced me to admit myself to a psychiatric ward. Otherwise, they warned, I could be admitted involuntarily. They worried I might become a danger to myself.

I was 49 years old when I was diagnosed with bipolar disorder and hospitalized for mania.

It was only after my second hospitalization one and a half years later (this time for depression) that I began to talk with colleagues about my diagnosis. Earlier that year I'd been out with a herniated disc, and when I returned to work many asked if my disc was acting up again. "No, it's not the disc," was my reply. "I'm bipolar and I was out with depression." At the time, my job involved consulting with nurses about difficult patients. After learning that I was bipolar, a few nurses stopped approaching me to discuss cases.

Examples like this make "coming out" as mentally ill an ongoing battle; I'm always afraid my career will be hurt by stereotypes and misconceptions. Bipolar disorder is a mood disorder; my intellect is not impaired. My days are not filled with dramatic highs and lows. In fact, my symptoms are well-controlled by medication and I work hard in therapy to avoid relapses. My husband attends therapy with me, and he can identify warning signs. For example, we both know that when I suddenly begin to sleep four instead of eight hours a night, it's time to visit my psychiatrist to have my medication adjusted.

Upon my first hospitalization I was handed a hospital gown and slippers and told to put all my clothing into a paper shopping bag. My purse and clothing were searched, and my husband was handed my nail clippers, file, and tweezers. He also took my wallet with my identification: I had become just a number on a wristband. But diligent attention to the requirements of my disorder has given me back my life. It's an opportunity that my mother and my colleague who committed suicide never had. I think my mother would be proud of what I've made of this chance. ▼

At Her Mercy

A nursing instructor finds herself in the hands of a challenging former student.

Alice C. Facente, MSN, RN-BC

I was having trouble breathing as I lay on that gurney in the chaotic ED. Was it a result of my fear? Or did I have an unseen pulmonary injury?

I had been in a car accident. I was in pain, and the cause of my pain was obvious. My neck hurt, my tibia poked through the skin on my right leg, and my right foot looked mangled and bloody. The reason for my fear was more complicated. Although I'd been a nurse for more than 20 years, this was the first time I had been so completely dependent on the health care system. I felt vulnerable. I knew too much. I needed to feel confident that the ED nurse assessing my injuries would do a thorough job and give unqualified support to a fellow nurse-turned-patient.

In walked the nurse who'd be caring for me. I stared at her. She looked familiar, like a slightly older version of a student I'd taught in the past. Even though the movement of my neck was restricted by a cervical collar, placed there by the emergency medical technician who brought me to the ED by ambulance, I managed to glance at her name tag. It was indeed Angela.

My mind raced back five years. It was my first year of teaching. I had eight students in that first clinical rotation, and seven of them were anxious and hesitant to actually touch the patients. Angela was different—in fact, she was somewhat confrontational and challenging. I didn't doubt her comprehension of the pathophysiology of disease; she'd aced her written exams. But applying theory to practice requires patience and critical thinking. Angela had been impulsive and impatient. She didn't seem to realize how crucial a careful, comprehensive patient assessment could be.

Worse, Angela tended to brush aside my admonitions. Because the assessment parts of her care plans frequently lacked critical data, her nursing diagnoses and interventions were often incomplete. When I had my individual conference with her, I explained my concerns and reviewed my written evaluation, which specified where improvement was needed.

But Angela was unconvinced. She rolled her eyes when I urged her to slow down and take greater care with the vital nursing process. I overheard her telling one of her classmates, "She's always picking on me because I'm young and quick."

I felt that my concerns were valid, but I also questioned my competence as a first-year instructor. Should I pass her? Or should I fail her, which would ultimately result in her expulsion from the nursing program? I slept poorly for several nights as I weighed the options. I consulted a faculty colleague who had similar concerns about Angela. I didn't want to be responsible for passing a student who'd be impetuous and careless—the results could be devastating. At the same time, I felt Angela could become an excellent nurse—she certainly had the potential. But passing or failing her was my call. Nursing students are truly at the mercy of their clinical instructors.

And now I was at *her* mercy. I had to put my trust completely in Angela. I asked if she remembered me. She laughed as she said, "Of course. How could I forget you?"

Her response only in creased my apprehension. But she had a calm, soothing voice, and she was careful and deliberate as she began her assessment, proceeding from head to toe as I had taught her. I began to feel slightly more confident. As she systematically auscultated all of my lung fields, she asked, "Does this hurt? Can you take a deep breath?" She gently, skillfully palpated every inch of my abdomen, asking, "Does that hurt? How about this?" By the end of her assessment, I felt she'd become an astute and precise clinician. I heard her quietly give a comprehensive evaluation of my condition to the ED physician.

Angela came to see me in my hospital room after I was admitted. We talked for quite a while. She told me that I'd given her a wake-up call during that first clinical rotation. She really had listened to my warnings and admonitions and had begun to exercise more careful judgment. She said it took her a while to overcome her resentment of my criticism but later came to realize the value of that clinical experience. (Luckily, my accident occurred after she came to that realization!) Angela had matured into the kind of nurse I'd suspected she was capable of becoming five years earlier. I'd taken a calculated risk. What a relief to realize that giving her that passing grade was indeed the right call. ▼

Big Love

How "the baby" became "my son."

Marcia Gardner, MA, RN, CPNP, CPN

W e named our first child Robbie, after my father, who died when I was in high school. I was 31 years old when Robbie was born. Although my pregnancy was completely normal, I never went into labor. By the time the obstetrician decided to induce labor, I was more than 42 weeks into my pregnancy.

We'd planned on a typical, long, epidural-supported first labor, but a good situation quickly turned bad. Late decelerations, decreased variability, decreased movement, and meconium in the amniotic fluid—they all happened so fast that I barely had time to grasp the need for all the associated interventions. In the end, I underwent an emergency C-section.

When I awoke in the recovery room, with my abdominal incision burning, I learned Robbie weighed slightly more than 5 lbs. Three weeks earlier, his estimated weight had been more than 8 lbs. Meetings with neonatologists began. Conversations were laden with laboratory data. "The baby," as they called him, had a decreased white cell count. A serious infection. Thrombocytopenia. Pneumothorax. "The baby" needed head ultrasonography and could have developmental problems in the future.

I was bombarded with so much information, such a multitude of potential problems, and was spending so little time with my newborn son that after two days he was beginning to sound like nothing more than a complex set of medical conditions.

My loved ones could offer me no reprieve. My husband, focused on the joy of a newborn son, didn't grasp the potential long-term implications of Robbie's problems. My mother searched for reasons for his condition, concluding that it was my fault for working too hard and having pets in the house while pregnant. Conversations with my siblings can be summed up as: "My friend had a baby who was little and that baby turned out great."

It was Robbie's nurses who helped me see beyond his medical challenges. They congratulated me on the birth of a sweet and beautiful baby boy, which no one else had done. They hurried into my room as his physicians hurried out saying "we don't know yet." They stayed with me as I cried. The nurses called him Robbie, not "the baby." They pointed out my son's miniature hands and complimented me on his long fingers. They admired his huge, clear blue eyes, his soft baby hair, and his big gummy smile. They reassured me that there was a lot that was baby-like, not diseaselike, about him.

After five days I was discharged, and Robbie was moved to the transitional nursery. The medical staff continued to test his blood and give him ultrasonography, X-rays, and hip evaluations. I visited every day, hearing results of each and every new test given to "the baby" as I sat by my son's bassinet.

Rita, the nurse in the transitional nursery, never left my side when I needed her, always making time to listen to my worries. When I came to visit, she told me Robbie was "such a cute little guy" and had "such a big personality." She picked him up and slung him over her shoulder, showing me that he was strong. She held him upright and spoke straight to his face. "You fresh little guy," she scolded, her voice warm and teasing. "You're giving your mom a lot of grief."

Just out of school, I'd worked in a level III neonatal intensive care unit. At 22 years old, I made a point of finding beautiful features in every tiny newborn face and of showing mothers that their babies, although vulnerable, were also strong and could be handled, held, and hugged. But I'd done so because that's what the literature and my teachers had instructed me to do. It was only when I became a mother that I truly understood the power of our words and deeds.

Nine days after Robbie was born, as I finally headed home with my son, I looked back at Rita. She nodded, smiling, as though she knew that we were ready to take this step and that we would thrive. And we did. Robbie is 15 years old now and he plays the piano beautifully (those nurses were right about his fingers), including a particularly memorable version of Fleetwood Mac's "Big Love." ▼

A Mind in Search of Its Moorings

Postsurgical psychosis in older adults is not uncommon, but that doesn't make it easy.

Jean DiMotto, JD, MSN, RN

An anesthesiologist was visiting with me three weeks after my surgery for bladder cancer. During that eight-hour operation, my bladder and gallbladder (with its gallstones) were removed, severe scarring and adhesions were lysed, a urostomy was created, and a mesh was sewn into place to repair my abdominal wall hernia. My postoperative course was also complicated.

"There are so many ways to be sick," the anesthesiologist commented. One of them is mental. After spending 10 of 21 days in a windowless ICU room, suffering the impact of all that was done to me in surgery and the ICU, and experiencing my physiology in tumult, I was mentally injured.

There was a large, round clock in each room that provided the time but not whether it was AM or PM. Once, a team of four came into my ICU room. The woman on the team said, "Good morning." Her greeting caught my attention. I was intubated, so I did my best to look intently at her and then at the clock, back to her, back to the clock. Fortunately, she understood. "Yes, it *is* morning." Ah, a simple certainty in a 24/7 environment.

In addition, just the numerical date was written on a whiteboard, but there was no calendar to provide a visual context for the date in the month.

To relieve excruciating postoperative pain, my pain management team put me under conscious sedation for four days. During and subsequent to these days I had phantasmagorical waking dreams. In one, I thought I was at an exclusive birthday party for a wealthy man, and I asked my husband and the respiratory therapist if our being right outside the party room was interfering with the party.

This continued on the step-down unit. Because I was sedated, I didn't experience the transfer between units. So I simply woke up in a new room. But I was dreaming vividly, as well as hallucinating, and thought I was in one of five different rooms.

I dreamt my daytime experiences. Seven days of arm restraints in the ICU because of the endotracheal tube? I dreamt of being restrained in bed for hours in a large room with others who were similarly restrained. Electrocautery in surgery? I dreamt of a man in blue scrubs using some type of electric gun on me.

My experiences were symptomatic of ICU psychosis. My physicians diagnosed delirium and attributed it to the pain medications and an abdominal infection; nonetheless, they also ordered neurology and psychology consults as well as an EEG and a CT scan of my brain. No functional defect was found—just a mind in search of its moorings.

My first conscious awareness that something was amiss was when a nurse began quizzing me about whether I knew where I was. Uh-oh. She repeated the question three or four times, then switched to, "Are you at home?" Phew! A clue. "No." "Where are you?" she repeated several more times. Finally, I figured out I was in the hospital. "Which one?" Oh no! Right answers are bad; they bring more questions! I gave an incorrect answer based on one of my dreams.

Since my surgery had taken place in early January, I had not yet internalized the change in the year and consistently got that answer wrong, although I finally put together that it was still January, not February, because the Super Bowl had not yet been played. As to the president's name, I just gave a name of any president during whose term I have lived. Where my many birth dates came from I will never know.

My husband and daughter observed these little sessions. While at times amused, they were also worried. I wish someone had reassured them that this was a not-uncommon, temporary occurrence in a 60-year-old after major surgery and its sequelae.

It took longer than my three-week hospitalization to come to terms with the fact that what I thought had been reality was in fact dream based. Even six weeks after discharge I was asking my husband whether something had actually happened. He had been with me in the hospital 21 hours a day, so he was an excellent resource for these reality checks.

Healing of the mind is subtle and takes time. It cannot be focused on—the mind prefers to be left to its own devices as it heals. There are no exercises with 10 reps each, no special foods.

I did notice improvement when I concentrated over the course of two weeks on filling in the blanks (e-mail addresses, etc.) in my cell phone "Contacts" list, adding missing contacts, and proofreading the changes. Twelve weeks after surgery, I was able to journal again. But it took a full four months before my mind had healed enough that I could return to my intellectual work as a judge. ▼

The Other Cancer Story

Is this a breast cancer competition?

Suellen Hozman, BS, RN

The audience huddles at round tables in the big room. The tables are set; there are cloth napkins. There's a raised platform for the speakers and fundraisers. Then it begins. Quiche, fruit, and pep talks. First, the executive director of Making Strides Against Breast Cancer gives the I'm-so-moved-at-the-outpouring-of-support speech. Next, time is given to the businesses that pledged the largest amount of money to the organization. You'd recognize the names. They're the big employers in your community. Finally, there is the survivor.

She is upbeat, grateful, and hopeful—despite the chemo, radiation, and surgery. She's in her 30s. She has small children. She smiles when she describes how much she loves her doctors and nurses. She says that she's a better person now. She doesn't describe the indigestible images of cancer: nonanesthetized injections at the tumor site, breasts and nipples inflamed from radiation. The audience finds her inspiring; their quiche goes down just fine.

I admire the survivor. I'm happy for her strength and spirit. I feel terrible that she got breast cancer at such a young age, before her children were grown. As a single parent, I asked not to die until my boys were grown. I got that wish.

But there's another side to the cancer story.

I joined the club on May 8, 2000. I was at my mother's apartment when I called my doctor's office for my results. I was shocked. So was my mother. "And you eat vegetables," she said. "You never know." At 86, a first-generation American born of Russian Jewish parents, my mother knew something about life's absence of guarantees.

From the beginning, my close friends and immediate family were wonderful. After the diagnosis, my good friend Robert drove me to my son Joshua's house. Joshua, who fills a doorway, held me, wept, and said, "Mom, we're doing this together."

But it was different with acquaintances. With them, conversations would go like this:

"I have breast cancer."

"Oh, I know an aunt [sister, wife, friend, coworker] who had breast cancer."

How should I have responded? Need I have asked to hear their stories and braced myself to learn about the dead ones? Is this a breast cancer competition? I wanted to ask, "Do you want me to feel good about my diagnosis just because I'm still alive?" It stunned me that coworkers and acquaintances found it so hard to simply listen. Why was it so uncommon for someone to say, "I'm sorry for your pain"?

I tried a local support group. The stories from the young women dealing with second and third occurrences were too brutal. It reminded me of my childhood neighbors, Holocaust survivors with numbers on their arms. It felt like breast cancer genocide. I made it to only one meeting.

So I became private, no longer sharing my diagnosis in casual interactions. I needed all my emotional reserves to survive the damn treatments. The cancer never hurt until I agreed to get cured.

There's no cookie-cutter treatment for breast cancer. Mine was mine: two surgeries, six weeks of radiation, and 13 months of tamoxifen (Nolvadex). It caused vocal chord disturbance, resurrection of irritable bowel syndrome, first-ever asthma symptoms, nonstop vaginal yeast infections, and atrophic vaginitis. Tamoxifen was killing me. But no alternate drug options were made available, even after I asked my oncologist. So I simply stopped taking it.

But I never stopped working. I received radiation at 7:15 AM and was usually at work by 8. No one brought me food, mowed my lawn, offered to take me out, or brought me a candle. As a single parent since 1978, I've come to be known as independent and self-sufficient. I didn't ask for help; I just continued on, day by day. There are millions like me out there who didn't win the Tour de France after cancer.

So I'm not a better person as a result of cancer. I'm unattractively hypochondriacal. I feel a pain in my groin after my daily walk and wonder if it's the first sign of pelvic cancer. Cancer wasn't my epiphany. It was painful and lonely. I'm the other cancer story. And I'm still alive. ▼

The Enduring Self

Living with mental illness can teach a nurse to see beyond a person's symptoms.

Marilyn Wargo, BSN, RNC

I am bipolar. I'm unable to get life insurance. That still shocks me, but I understand the reason. Suicide is always a possibility in mental illness, and during the darkest episode of my illness, I almost attempted it. Remembering that period of my life, although it was 30 years ago, is still painful. But I'm a better nurse for having learned to live with chronic illness. It has helped me to understand my patients as people and see beyond their diagnosis.

My attempt at suicide followed the death of my second child, Loura Michelle, who coded right after birth and died four hours later of what was determined to be polycystic kidney disease. A few weeks later we moved into a new home. No one noticed that I wasn't sleeping at all. I was caring for our two-year-old while trying to set up the home without the baby we had enthusiastically awaited to make it complete. I kept hauling the same boxes from room to room but couldn't decide where to put anything. This unproductive frenzy was my way of escaping painful thoughts of our loss. Soon, my mind began to create its own reality. One day, in the grip of a hallucination, I found myself sitting in the living room telling my husband and his relatives what the Holy Spirit wanted them to know. My husband interrupted to say he was taking me to the hospital. Grabbing my maternity bras with other clothes made perfect sense to me: my husband was taking me to the psychiatric unit, but in my mind I was going to the hospital to get my baby back.

The intern working with my psychiatrist asked a lot of questions, trying to assess my mental state. I was a staff nurse at the hospital and we knew each other as colleagues. Just four weeks before, I'd performed a code in the ICU with this man. I can imagine how I must have looked to him—clothes awry, no makeup, hair uncombed.

That night when my husband brought our little girl to visit, I resolved to get out of there. The next morning, I craftily asked my doctor what I needed to do to be well. He said that if I could concentrate enough to read a book or accomplish other tasks, it would be evidence of improvement. I immediately set about performing, as if according to script—making my bed, watching television, reading an article—to earn his approval for discharge. The strategy worked. My husband drove me home and sleeping pills knocked me out that night, but the world I woke up to was not one that others shared.

We've all seen the elegant coronet of a splashing drop, captured in photographs that seem to make time stand still. I felt frozen in time like one of those drops. The second hand of the clock in our living room took an eternity to move one tick, and I found myself waiting for the next tick as if this was all there was to life. Desperate to escape, I went outside and headed for the cars rushing along a highway near my house. I was only 20 ft. from throwing myself onto the highway when I heard my little girl yelling, "Mommy, I want to go with you." I turned to catch her and started to cry.

I was locked in my hospital's suicide-prevention unit and heavily medicated. Some of the medications made my gait unsteady; others made me faint. After two weeks I was allowed to go home on antidepressants. Even so, the depressive episode lasted a year. My physicians initially thought I was suffering from postpartum depression or an overwhelming grief reaction. Eventually, I was diagnosed with bipolar disorder and started on lithium. In the years since, I've had a few breakdowns, but never as serious as that first one, even after I lost a second baby to polycystic disease.

Just because I'm on medication for my illness doesn't mean I'm not able to perform professionally. I'm blessed with an optimistic husband, an extensive support network of friends and family, good psychiatric care, and effective medication. My spiritual life also is strong, and it helps me through.

In the three decades since I was diagnosed with bipolar disorder, I have learned that I am much more than my illness. This perspective, though it came at a price, is valuable for me as a nurse. I see my patients in the throes of acute episodes of disease or debilitated by amyotrophic lateral sclerosis or Parkinson disease and understand perfectly when they insist that this is not who they really are. ▼

The Sacraments of Sister Thecla

Principles and Practices of Nursing.

Madeleine Mysko, MA, RN

When I was a nursing student, back in the late '60s, Principles and Practices of Nursing was held in a dim classroom on the first floor of our nurses' residence. There the freshman students would sit in the old, theater-style tiers, intent on the instructions of Sister Thecla.

Sister Thecla was tall, thin, and slightly stooped. We "girls" were only 18, and thought she was old. But now it occurs to me that her posture probably reflected humility—or perhaps the discomfort of shyness—more than it did her age. Her voice quavered a bit, like that of a maiden great-aunt. Her face wore an expression of continual, mild concern. She wasn't one of those nuns whose gaze you feared. Sister Thecla's pale eyes were often looking away, or down at her spotless shoes.

Sister Thecla taught us that nursing was "an art and a science." She taught us the proper order of the full bed bath, the modesties of the "local bath," the imperatives of the back rub, and the refinements of the draw-sheet, the emesis basin, and the ordinary washcloth. She demonstrated that the art and science of nursing required all the scrupulous attentions to detail of a priest celebrating High Mass.

At the center of Sister Thecla's demonstrations was an old manikin that lived all its days on the hospital bed at the front of the classroom. I can still see its chipped, painted face—the trust in the eyes, the unreadable thin lips. I can see Sister Thecla turning that manikin on its side, taking care so the blanket wouldn't slip and expose any imagined privates. And Sister Thecla's hands—how they were all tenderness, and how somehow, right before our eyes, they transubstantiated the cotton backside of that manikin into the feverish, aching flesh of a real sick person.

The other night, Sister Thecla visited me in a dream. I hadn't thought of her in years, and yet there she was. I don't know how to describe the power of this dream, except to say that I can't seem to let it go.

Right before this dream, I'd been admitted to the hospital, by way of the ED, after a bout of chest pain that radiated up into my throat. The pain had come out of the blue, so of course it was a scare. But by the time I'd scooted myself from the gurney and into a bed on the unit—where they'd watch over me until the stress test in the morning—the pain was gone, and the blood work had come back negative.

The nurse was kind and efficient. After she'd gone over me thoroughly, she wrote her beeper and cell phone numbers on the board at the foot of my bed. She encouraged me to call any time. "For anything at all," she said, smiling. "Really, anything." And then she was gone.

I wasn't afraid. And except for the unwieldiness of being attached to a monitor and iv tubing, I wasn't uncomfortable. Though I'd been cautioned not to eat or drink, in truth I wasn't even hungry. The room was semiprivate, but the other bed was empty. It was the end of the evening shift.

A friendly nursing assistant came to take my vital signs. When I almost made the mistake of saying that the unit seemed quiet, she shushed me: "No, no, don't say that word." I laughed and told her I was a nurse myself and understood all about jinxes. I settled down then under the extra bath blankets she'd brought me. She turned out the lights.

I wasn't afraid, and yet, suddenly and inexplicably, I felt as though my heart had been broken. I felt abandoned, by whom I couldn't say. The tears ran down my face into the stiff pillowcase. I had such a lump in my throat—real pressure—that I was afraid something would show on the monitor.

This is nonsense, I told myself. *Get to sleep.*

Somehow I did.

And then she came to me: Sister Thecla, carrying her old porcelain basin, the linens, the lotions and powder. She turned me on my side, her arms stronger than I'd ever imagined they'd be. Her hands moved slowly down the length of my spine, kneading in tenderness. *It isn't nonsense*, she said, leaning close. *You know that.* She made a gentle sound, a grandmotherly *tsk, tsk* close to my ear.

Oh my, she said close to my ear, in that quavering voice from long ago. *Whatever happened to PM care?* ▼

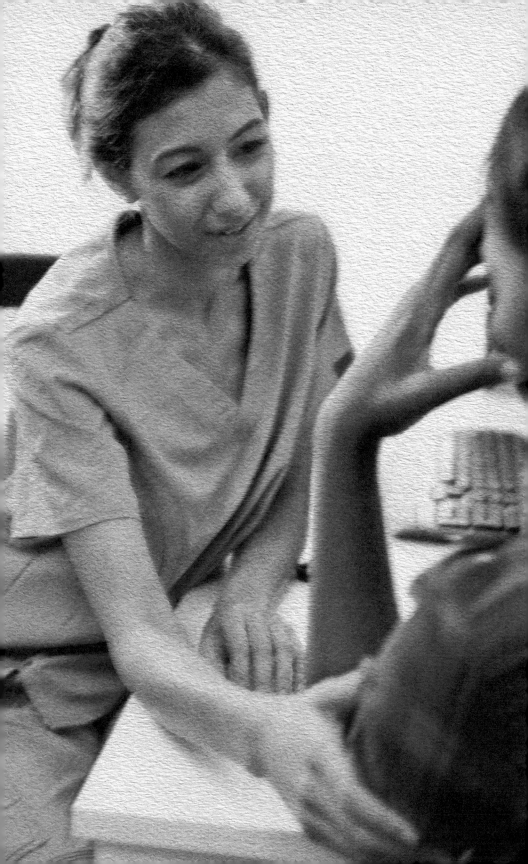

Making A Difference

Stories of nurses going above and beyond—just doing the simple things that make a difference in their patients' lives.

"But I do the only thing I can, the one thing I could promise. I stay with her."

Danielle Allen, RN

Am I Going to Be Okay?

Keeping the trust of patients at critical moments.

Danielle Allen, RN

A m I going to be okay?" Ami gasps. Her breath hitches, her chest rising and falling in spasms. One of my hands holds a mask to her face; the other hand holds hers. Pain has made her strong—my fingers are almost as white as her pale face, radiant with fear.

She's in danger—but I don't think she will die. The doctor is on her way and I think we can save Ami. But although nurses and physicians pride themselves on fixing people, Ami's life is about to change once again, and her future is uncertain.

Ami stares at me, her brown eyes like river pebbles as tears wash over them. I know she is waiting for my answer—so is her husband, standing behind me, watching as I crouch at her bedside.

My instinct is to tell them yes, everything is going to be okay. I don't want Ami to panic, and keeping her calm will help the outcome. But I also don't want to lie. During the last week, I've built a relationship of trust with Ami through patience and compassion, but most importantly, through honesty.

Ami has been in and out of hospitals her whole life. A genetic disease has committed her to frequent-flier status, and she has spent years of her young adult life struggling to breathe, eat, and live like a normal person. The accumulated pain and fear from her hospital stays seems to have manifested as severe anxiety and a desperate need for control.

Lying to Ami now would reinforce her feelings of mistrust for nurses and physicians, but I want to do it anyway. I want to tell her it will be okay, because I want it to be true. And I think she wants me to say it. She trusts me—if I promise it will be okay, she'll believe me. Then maybe she'll feel that this whole emergency will soon be over.

My mind returns to a time I'll never forget, when I heard a nurse tell a patient it would be okay. It was during a code. Blood sprayed with every heartbeat. While one nurse applied pressure, the primary nurse suctioned blood and kept repeating, "It's okay, you'll be okay," long after he'd lost consciousness.

I'm sure she didn't intend for the last thing he'd ever hear to be a lie. Probably, she was saying the only thing she thought might help. And who knows, she might not have even been talking to him, but to herself. "It's okay, you'll be okay" is many nurses' mantra in moments of stress—when a confused patient turns violent, when a frustrated staff member yells, when you've made a mistake.

Still, that moment sits like a rock on my heart. Should you tell a patient it will be okay, when you know it won't? Some patients find the phrase comforting, even when they know the prognosis is bleak. Others may lose trust. As a health care provider, it can be difficult to guess how these common words of comfort will be received. And if you don't say it will be okay, what *do* you say? I want my patients to trust me, but I also want them to feel safe and reassured. Where's the line?

I look into Ami's wide eyes, dilated with panic. She's desperate for me to answer her question.

I open my mouth to lie, but different words come out. "I don't know exactly what will happen, but I'll stay with you."

Ami closes her eyes and lays her head back on the pillow. Tendrils of wet hair cling to her gown. I don't know if her hair is wet from tears, or from when I helped her wash her hair in the sink this morning. That feels like a long time ago now.

Every word is a struggle for Ami, but she forces them out. "The last time I asked a nurse if I'd be okay, she said yes. But I wasn't." Ami turns to me. "Thank you for not lying to me."

Her grip loosens on my hand, so I squeeze it gently.

"Can we breathe together?" I ask.

Ami nods. We did this earlier today when she struggled to catch her breath. In slowly through the nose, visualizing the lungs inflating like a balloon. Out slowly through the mouth, like blowing through a straw.

"In," I say, and our lungs open together. "Out," I say, and we both release.

In, out. In, out. In, out.

Ami's breath is slower, almost comfortable for the first time since the emergency started. Still, it will probably not be okay.

But I do the only thing I can, the one thing I could promise.

I stay with her. ▼

Socks and All...

An OR nurse opts for empathy and honesty in responding to an adolescent patient's fears.

Bryanne Hickey Harrington, BSN, RN, CNOR

As the circulating nurse in our busy OR that Friday, I went to pre-op our last case: "Katie," a 14-year-old who'd been diagnosed with multiple osteochondromas. These tumors are typically composed of bony fibers and cartilage. They're usually benign but can cause pain. On several occasions Katie had come to the ED with pain so severe she'd vomited. She needed OxyContin to sleep at night and had stopped going to school. The lesion on the underside of her left arm was so painful she couldn't even brush her hair. A larger lesion on the inner aspect of her scapula caused searing chest pain when she took a deep breath. She'd seen a neurologist, psychologists, the pain service, and finally our orthopedist, who would remove the lesions and give her back her life.

We were preparing the OR when the pre-op nurse called to say Katie had locked herself in the bathroom and was crying uncontrollably. Her mother was trying to talk to her through the door. The problem was that Katie didn't want to remove her bra—didn't want any men to see her naked. Her mother wanted us to lie and say that the bra would stay on.

As a rule, an OR nurse's job is very technical; we interact with patients and their families only briefly. Before the operation we quickly assess the patient and ensure that she or he is prepared for surgery. We introduce ourselves, then check and double-check documents and lab results. Patients don't often remember the nurses who hold their hands as they go under anesthesia, nor do they realize that those nurses pride themselves on being the patients' advocate while they're asleep.

In the case of a pediatric patient, a parent or guardian signs the consent forms. But if a child voices strong opposition to surgery, it's the OR nurse's ethical responsibility to investigate the concern. And so I assured Katie's mother that we'd take excellent care of her daughter, but that I'd want to be honest in speaking to Katie.

I had to introduce myself to Katie through the bathroom door. Once she let me in, I gave her a tissue and asked her to sit down and take a deep breath. I told her I'd explain everything that was going to happen from the time we left the pre-op area, and that it was my job to keep her safe through her surgery. I said I'd answer her questions. I said I wanted her to feel comfortable with the plan before we went ahead.

Katie responded that she wouldn't take off her bra and didn't want anyone to see her naked. As I crouched in front of her, I thought how much easier it would be to do as her mother had asked and just lie. But I knew this would violate Katie's modesty, and the trust she'd just put in me. I didn't want to fuel a distrust of those who'd care for her in the future. And I remembered how difficult it was to be 14, with raging emotions and a changing body.

So I told Katie the truth: eventually, the bra had to come off.

At first, she seemed even more upset. But then I told her I'd be the one to take the bra off after she was asleep—the one keeping her covered, making sure only those who needed to be there were there. I promised to treat her like I'd want to be treated myself. And that all this would be worth it to not have the horrible pain.

Katie was still crying when I said the surgeon would be coming to see her in a few minutes. I told her I'd watch the bathroom door from the outside if she kept it unlocked. I told her to think about what I'd said. Then I went to inform the attending surgeon about the mother's concerns and Katie's wishes.

At last, Katie emerged from the bathroom, her eyes swollen, nose dripping. She said she'd do it if it would happen as I told her it would.

We proceeded. After several hours, two osteochondromas the size of golf balls had been removed. Before Katie woke up, I redressed her—socks and all—and wheeled her to the postanesthesia area. I went to visit her that following Monday. She told me she was embarrassed that she'd cried but was glad I'd told her the truth.

In the perioperative area it's easy to forget the value of simple actions like preserving the modesty of our patients. But on this day, communicating honestly with my patient paved the way for a successful surgery. ▼

A Change of Heart

A lasting payoff for the long shifts and lost personal time.

Nancy Cabianca, RN

I've been a nurse for more than half of my life. I've worked in many areas, from neonatal, pediatric, and adult ICUs to emergency and operating rooms. I've worked in hospitals, physician's offices, and long-term care facilities. I love my career and consider myself blessed to have found my calling. But we all experience times when our long hours and the rigorous demands of this job make us feel that we sacrifice too much of our personal and family time to care for strangers.

I had this feeling one Christmas Day a few years ago. I had been working my regular eight-hour shift, six-in-a-row stretch, with Christmas Eve, Christmas Day, and Boxing Day right at the end. I was in charge for the stretch and also was covering "on call for hearts" for three of the six shifts. I was low enough on the seniority roster that, for the third year in a row, I couldn't get any time off for the holidays, though at least this year it was day shifts instead of nights.

On Christmas Day, we had four back-to-back emergency CABGs starting at 8 AM and stretching long past my scheduled 3 PM end of shift. I had called in the on-call team for a C-section at 8 AM, and they had stayed all day doing emergency cases as well. Our two teams saw each other as we passed in the hallway, wishing "Merry Christmas" as we rolled our patients to and from the ORs. I called home several times that day to tell my husband not to wait for me, to go visit his family without me, to eat without me, and then to go home without me. Each time we were in the middle of one case we would get word that another was waiting. Finally, I told my husband not to wait up for me. I had missed another Christmas with my family.

At 10 minutes before midnight, the circulator wheeled our second heart transplant patient into the OR. He looked over at me behind the huge back table that I was setting up with all the instruments and gadgets required to perform the small miracle that is a heart transplant. I gave him a wave and reassured him that I was getting everything ready for him. He smiled, pointed to his head, and in a heavy French-Canadian accent, said "pumpkin."

I knew what he meant. He was referring to my brightly colored hat. It was my habit to wear a red hat whenever I worked in the heart rooms.

I corrected him: "Not pumpkin... tomato." He smiled, nodding in agreement. Looking at the clock, I remarked that he must have been a very good boy this year for Santa to bring him a new heart. He started to cry.

"You know," he said, "I told my family today that this will be my last Christmas with them."

I stopped my busy hands and listened.

"I have been sick so long, and felt so bad for so long, and have been waiting for a heart for so long. I gave up hope. I told them that I cannot go on much longer feeling this bad. I told them that I will die soon."

I felt my throat get tight, my eyes fill with water. He looked so frail and tired. He sobbed, wiping his tears with the bedsheet.

"And then we got the call that you have my heart. Thank you. Thank you for being here in the middle of this Christmas night away from your family to do this for me. You are away from your family because of me," he sobbed.

The circulating nurse put her arms around him and held him. "We are here *for* you, not *because* of you," she said.

The surgery went smoothly. Our patient received his new heart and was sent to post-op, still asleep and on the ventilator. We still had one more heart transplant to do. I left to go home at around 4 AM.

On Boxing Day, I came back to work. I never go to see our patients in the cardiac surgical ICU. Patients don't often remember nurses from the OR, and I don't want to make them feel uncomfortable or to intrude on them in any way. But on this day, at the end of my shift, I went in search of my French-Canadian patient.

He was right there as soon as I entered—awake, sitting up in bed, and off the ventilator. I was startled that he looked so great. He spotted me, pointed to his head, and mouthed "pumpkin." I corrected him: "Not pumpkin. Tomato."

He motioned for me to come closer, clasped my hand, and whispered, "I can never thank you enough for this gift you have given me." I held his hand tighter and whispered, "Me neither." ▼

A Brief Respite

When a family is wounded.

Kelly Carroll, BA, RN

Sliding my stethoscope beneath the fold of his hospital gown, I listened to the boy's heart. It was before 8 AM and his room was still dark, yet there was something striking about his stillness. He didn't jump at the initial touch of the stethoscope as other five-year-olds would. Instead, he continued sleeping, not reacting to the strange room, my presence, or the unexpected cool metal on his skin. Was his stillness caused by profound exhaustion, medication, or something else? Jonathan had been hit by a car the day before and had sustained a broken leg and slight bruising on his face. I wondered: What allows a child to find such respite in the dissonant rings and beeps of a hospital?

Jonathan had been home alone with his younger brother when the accident happened. The Department of Children and Families had been called to investigate the possibility of child neglect. His mother, Theresa Evans, was slumped on the foldout couch next to his bed; she remained asleep as I checked on her son.

When I came back into the room about an hour later, Ms. Evans asked me about getting a breakfast tray. I was fairly new to the facility and didn't know the protocol, so I told her I would find out if they were available for family members. She then became agitated. "If you think I'm going to stay with him," she said, pointing to her son, "all day here in this hospital, you're wrong." Jonathan was awake; I looked into his eyes and he held my gaze. He had the look of someone who has long since passed the point of asking for help. It was an expression that should never find its way to the face of a child. I felt my throat burn and I swallowed, deciding simply to do what I could to get what Ms. Evans needed.

I left to make peanut butter sandwiches. When I returned, Ms. Evans wouldn't look at me. "He won't eat this," was her only response. She wore a stained and ill-fitting fast-food-chain–employee shirt. Her hair was uneven and fell in her face; it was dirtier than expected after one night's stay in the hospital. I wondered where her family was, the boy's father. She hadn't used the phone since arriving at the hospital, and no one came to visit the boy that day. Worried that I would upset her further, I didn't ask her the whereabouts of her other son. She ate her sandwich hungrily and quickly, not stopping to acknowledge anyone else in the room. Jonathan accepted his sandwich and chewed it slowly.

Despite her initial assertion, Ms. Evans stayed at the hospital, missing a full day of work. She seemed to embrace the role of Jonathan's protector and caregiver. She attended to her son, beginning to accept help, warily, from those of us ducking in and out of the room. She seemed to act instinctively—at one moment confrontational, and the next protective.

As the day wore on, Ms. Evans was interviewed by the hospital's pediatrician, investigators from the Department of Children and Families, and social services. When the influx subsided, I asked about bathing Jonathan. I was sure she was raw from the questions about her parenting skills. "Could you do it?" she asked, her voice flat, without feeling. "I just don't know what to do with the cast or all the wires and cords." I told her I'd be happy to, adding that bathing could be difficult with all these new things hooked up.

As we busied ourselves caring for Jonathan, I began to joke with him and then, gingerly, with Ms. Evans. "He likes to do things himself, doesn't mind getting messy," she said. "Look what he's done with the paints! He's covered in them." The Child Life Department had given him paints and a small treasure box, and he was busily painting in bed, the lively colors marking his hands, face, even the bright white of his new cast. I laughed. "The cast looks truly personalized with all this color," I told him. "Very creative!" Ms. Evans smiled. "He can do all kinds of things," she replied. Her eyes followed his brush as he smeared paint across the wooden box. I told her he seemed like a strong boy, with plenty of interests. She nodded. I began to sense her own relief at being in the hospital; it mirrored that of her son's, as if she had finally been discovered, accused, and saved all in one day. ▼

May I Have a Band-Aid?

When a bandage can't cover the wound.

Marie F. Kerscher, BEd, RN and Coordinated by Veneta Masson, MA, RN

Being the sole health care provider at a busy urban high school of 1,500 students presents daily challenges. I see 50 to 80 students a day for all sorts of things, from sickle cell anemia, diabetes, and seizure disorders, to pregnancy, trauma, and malingering.

When Marcus first came to see me, I was sitting at my desk trying to catch up on some paperwork. He stood in my doorway and asked, "May I have a Band-Aid?" Such a request is not unusual, so I handed him one and turned back to my work.

"May I have a larger Band-Aid?" he asked. I handed him a larger one.

Several moments went by. He was still standing there in the doorway, silent and staring at the floor. "Can I help you with something else?" I asked.

"Maybe you could look at this," he said, pointing to his upper arm.

A frayed dressing, the color of a dirty sweat sock, was wrapped around it.

"Why don't you tell me what's under this dressing?" I said as I began unwrapping the gauze.

"I was shot," he said softly, looking away.

"With a gun?" I asked, stunned.

"Yeah," he replied.

I closed my office door and sat next to him. "Will you tell me what happened?"

And so he explained, his gaze never meeting mine, that he and a friend had been in a minor car accident. They'd had an argument with the other driver, who had a gun. After the police arrived, Marcus was transported to the ED, where he was treated and given a prescription for antibiotics. The police had already been looking for Marcus, so they took him to the local youth detention center, where he remained for three days.

As I unwound the gauze, my thoughts whirled. I had never seen a gunshot wound. What would it look like? A small entry wound? A large exit wound? Would it be infected?

It was all of the above. I asked if he was taking the antibiotics. "No," he answered. "They didn't give me any pills." He reached into his pocket and pulled out a wrinkled wad of paper. "I have this," he said. Unfolding it carefully, I saw it was the prescription from the ED.

I needed to contact his parent or guardian. I called the numbers in Marcus's file. All of them were disconnected. I asked him if he knew of someone who might be able to help him—an aunt or uncle or grandparent—anybody.

After a pause, he answered, "I can't think of anyone."

We sat in silent discouragement, and I wondered what it must be like to be 15 and have nobody to call when you need help.

"Maybe you could try Joe," he said, and gave me the number of his mother's former boyfriend. Joe was home, and he assured me that he would get Marcus's prescription filled and buy supplies for the dressings. I asked Marcus to stop back the next day so I could check his arm. He smiled and looked me in the eye for the first time and said he would.

Marcus didn't come to school the next day. Or the day after that. But days later, a beaming Marcus appeared in my doorway holding a bulging brown paper sack. It was full of supplies: gauze squares, roller gauze, tape, and the antibiotics. He took each item out one by one to show me.

When he held out his arm so I could change his bandage, I saw the dirty, loose gauze I had applied the week before. I held up the bottle of antibiotics. "Marcus, have you taken any of your pills?"

Marcus shook his head. "I just got them today."

I watched him take two capsules and told him to come back at the end of the day for the second dose. Next, I told him exactly how to change his dressing and when to take the antibiotics. I wasn't sure when I'd see him again, so I made him repeat my instructions until I was certain he understood what to do.

Marcus left that day with a promise to return to my office on Monday.

But he didn't. It wasn't until four months later that Marcus came to see me again. The gunshot wound was completely healed. He had reestablished a relationship with his mother and was going to school in a different district.

During the months he was gone, I thought about him often. Students like Marcus come to see me every day. They're not worried about completing their homework; they're concerned with survival. What more can I do? Maybe it's enough to be here when they ask for a Band-Aid. ▼

The Dirtiest House in Town

Home care nursing isn't for the faint of heart.

Alice C. Facente, MSN, RN, BC

The convalescent-home referral said that Loretta was 71 years old with the usual health problems related to stroke and diabetes. It also said that her husband had a gun and "wasn't afraid to use it." Fiercely protective of his wife, he'd had many disputes with the nursing staff about her care. The discharge planner who'd referred her to our home care agency insisted that two nurses make the initial home visit.

When I arrived at the home, the admitting nurse was already in the driveway, embroiled in a discussion with the husband. Insisting that he'd take care of Loretta himself, he refused to allow us in the house. Although we told him that his wife's personal physician, whom he claimed to trust, had asked for our help, he remained adamant. Finally, after I said that we'd have to call 911 for a police escort, he let us in.

An overpowering odor of urine hit us as we entered the living room. We soon discovered it was from the couple's 14 cats and two dogs. The litter box was overflowing. It was so dark and dirty inside the house, we couldn't tell if the floor was linoleum or wood.

Loretta was sitting on the edge of a hospital bed in the living room, smiling. We introduced ourselves and told her we were there to take care of her. "I'm so happy to be home," she said, hugging her husband and two of the nearest cats. With her husband hovering nearby, we began a complete physical assessment.

Her husband had just filled all of her prescriptions and purchased an alternating air pressure mattress for the hospital bed, three sets of bed linens, pads for the bed, and an assortment of incontinence briefs.

We offered the services of Meals on Wheels, but he refused. The kitchen counters were grimy and cluttered. The kitchen sink was plugged, full of black, stagnant water and greasy pots. The only thing on the large wooden table was an aluminum baking pan filled with dry cat food. A cat lounged on every flat surface: the kitchen cabinets, counters, hospital bed, even the wheelchair. We didn't try to reason with the couple about sanitation issues surrounding these pets, at least not on this first visit.

We gave Loretta a sponge bath with her husband watching our every move. We taught him how to empty the urinary drainage bag and monitor her blood sugar, and instructed him on her medications, simplifying procedures wherever possible.

Each step of the way, we praised him for his fast learning. We told him we appreciated how devoted he was to Loretta, and that our goal was to help him continue to take good care of her. Loretta seemed oblivious to the dirty environment and her husband's intimidating manner, and accepted all of the care we provided.

By the time we were ready to leave, he hugged us, thanked us, and said we could come back anytime.

During my visit the next day, I convinced him to allow a home health aide to come and bathe Loretta. He agreed—but only if I made my nursing visits at the same time. When I arrived for the third visit, the husband showed me how he had unclogged the toilet, mopped the kitchen floor, and thrown all the dirty dishes in the garbage; he bought paper plates and plastic utensils to use.

The house never became what could be described as clean, but Loretta and her clothing always were. Loretta never developed pressure ulcers, pneumonia, or deep vein thrombosis. She had frequent urinary tract infections from the indwelling catheter, but her husband phoned me immediately when he recognized signs of infection, just as I had taught him.

At the end of every visit he always thanked me, and I never did see that legendary gun. ▼

What One Thing Will Make Today Better for You?

You never know what a patient really wants—unless you ask.

Susan L. Goff, MS, RN

It's been at least 10 years, but I still remember that it was a difficult morning getting to work. The snow was piled high and the roads weren't yet plowed. Nevertheless, all staff showed up—the usual when you worked on a busy oncology unit.

As nurse in charge of the unit, I received the night report from the off-going night nurse in charge. Mrs. Smith vomited for a good portion of the night; Mr. Jones's wife had to leave to go home and get the kids off to school—she was hoping to make it back "in time"; Mr. Ricker's wife stayed with him last night. She told me who was "critical," and what needs were primary in caring for each.

I made a round of the unit. As I walked into the patients' rooms, I greeted each with a touch on the hand or forehead and asked them, or their family if present, "What one thing would make today better for you?" I'd used this approach since the 1970s, when I'd realized that my assumptions about what mattered to patients were often incorrect.

The answers were always worth paying attention to. "Please turn off the light"; "please put another blanket on me"; "can I have some grapefruit juice?"; "when is my next pain medicine due and can I have it *now*?" All of these could be solved with a quick flick of the switch or pull of the blanket. A call to dietary directly from the room got the grapefruit juice within minutes, and a check of the med record directly outside the patient's room showed he was due for his medication and the nurse in charge of his care was on her way with it.

As I entered Mr. Ricker's room, I remembered that the night nurse had mentioned that his wife had been with him overnight. I knocked very lightly and opened the door a crack. The two of them were cuddled up closely in the bed. I asked quietly, "What one thing would make today better?" The answer came in a raspy whisper from Mr. Ricker: "rice pudding." Pondering the fact that he hadn't eaten in days, I said, "Let me work on that."

Mr. Ricker had been a patient on our unit for three weeks and was "actively dying." As I worked my way through the hallway, greeting family members and patients recovering enough to be up and about, I was preoccupied with his request.

Sure enough, when I checked the chart, his orders were NPO ("nothing by mouth"). I paged Dr. Miller; when I got his return call, I was ready for it. After hearing my request, he said, "Sue, are you crazy? I don't even know what pipes are connected to what since he's had so much surgery." I said I understood his concern, but that Mr. Ricker had requested the pudding and I'd really thought he looked much worse today. Couldn't we just try it, "even if we just let him put it in his mouth and taste it?" Dr. Miller's answer was a tentative "Well, all right." I thanked him and promised him I would have the suction ready and be available to assist his wife.

The next hurdle was to call dietary and find out if they even had rice pudding. They did. I told them the name and room number, but asked them to bring it to me at the nurses' station. I wanted to be sure I was present when the rice pudding arrived.

Then it was back to the work of the unit. After many phone calls and questions from physicians making rounds, the rice pudding was on the desk at the nurses' station in front of me. I'd consulted with Mr. Ricker's nurse and told her what was going on.

I brought the rice pudding to Mr. Ricker's room, knocked quietly, and entered. Again it was very quiet, with the two of them cuddled up in the bed. After a moment, his wife got up and took the rice pudding from me. Jim, in his raspy whisper, said, "Thanks Sue, you are the best." After she'd reassured me that she knew how to use the suction and would pull the emergency cord if she needed me, I left.

I remained outside the door with my ear to the door for several minutes, but I didn't hear a sound.

About an hour later, I checked back with Jim and his wife. Both were sleeping soundly. The empty rice pudding dish was on the bedside table.

That afternoon at about one o'clock, Jim died peacefully in his sleep with his wife cuddled up to him in the bed.

I never did find out who actually ate the rice pudding—Jim or his wife. ▼

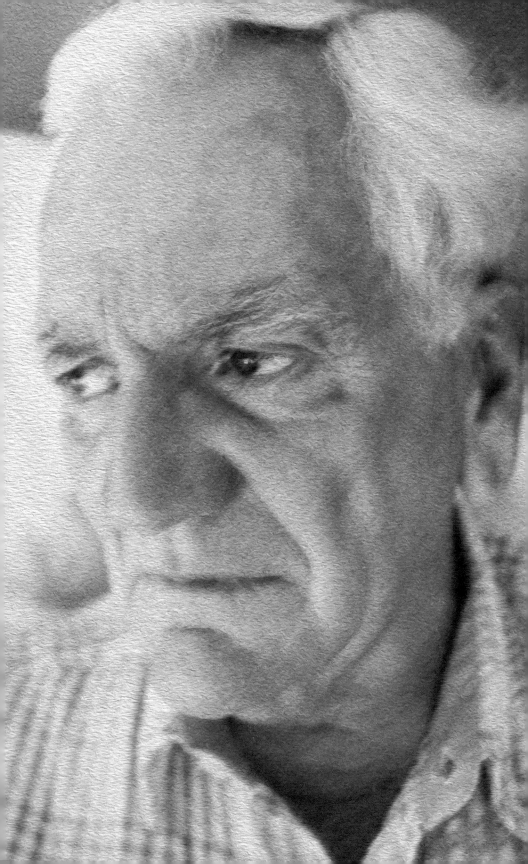

Memorable Patients

Stories of nurses caring for the difficult patients who test their patience and make them question their resolve or challenge them to find new insights, new solutions. And the inspiring patients that help them remember why they became a nurse.

"I could not have told him that I loved my job, that it was never dull, that it provided moments of odd intimacy like this one, that it gave pleasure in knowing what a nurse usually knows – that he or she is almost always of use."

Claire Brown, BSN, RN

Hiding a Tender Soul

A cold day on the waterfront, a nurse, a homeless man, and a canary yellow coat.

Cheryl Kane, MEd, BSN, RN

Patrick had once been a fisherman, living in Boston's North End, a predominantly Italian neighborhood until the young professionals moved in and many old-timers moved out. He had been married and gainfully employed before his life spiraled out of control and his low self-esteem, gambling, and drinking resulted in divorce and homelessness.

Patrick was disheveled, dirty, alcoholic, and feisty, although he could be a real charmer. Seventy years old, he was slight of build with a ruddy complexion, a bushy gray beard, and long, dirty fingernails.

Patrick hung out near the New England Aquarium next to the harbor. He spent his days stemming—street slang for panhandling. In the evening, he slept between Jersey barriers on a busy street that traces the shape of Boston's shoreline. In cold weather, he would wrap himself in the dark gray, felt-like blankets homeless advocates hand out when the temperatures drop.

As a member of the Boston Health Care for the Homeless Program's street team, I had been his nurse for several years. I knew the outlines of his early life: his mother died young; his stepmother rejected him. He often talked about killing himself. I once asked Patrick if he was scared to die and he told me that even God wouldn't want him. He rarely accepted health care from our team, but occasionally would allow us to take him back to one of the shelters for a shower and change of clothes.

One fall day, Patrick had been lying on a wall that ran along Boston Harbor when a friend pushed him into the water. He suffered a massive coronary and was hospitalized. A few weeks later I got a page from the local hospital, saying Patrick had left the hospital against doctor's orders, wearing only a hospital johnny and a vest.

It was an unusually cold Sunday in October. I rushed out to look for him. I wasn't surprised to find him in his usual spot between the Jersey barriers, swathed in blankets. I led him across the street and asked him to wait in front of the Dunkin' Donuts while I went to get him some clothes. When I returned with a set of men's clothes and a canary yellow down jacket, Patrick looked at me, then glanced disdainfully at the jacket and said that if he wore it, he would stick out like a sore thumb. He asked me where in the world I had gotten it.

I told him that it had belonged to my husband, Jim. When he asked me if he no longer wanted it, I told him Jim had died two years ago and would have been very happy for him to use it. Patrick's demeanor softened. "Oh, honey. I'm so sorry. Go into that Dunkin' Donuts, buy yourself a coffee—put it on my tab," he instructed. "Then come back and tell me all about your husband."

I went into Dunkin' Donuts and bought a coffee. I paid for it myself. When I returned, he invited me to sit on a milk crate and tell him about my husband. I told him how we hadn't been married for very long before Jim developed a brain tumor, how sick he had gotten, how he loved to run marathons. What I didn't tell Patrick was that our wedding anniversary was that weekend. It was always a difficult time of year for me. My moments of connection with Patrick made it a little easier.

That encounter with Patrick shaped my nursing practice. Working with long-term homeless people can be very challenging, physically and emotionally. Their lice-infested bodies can disconcert even the most experienced nurse. Cleaning them can take your breath away. They can be rejecting, belligerent, ungrateful.

Yet here was this homeless man who fit every stereotype, reaching out to me at a time when I was very vulnerable. His generous spirit and sensitivity taught me the importance of looking beyond the exterior. The tenderest of souls can be contained within the most unlikely of vessels. You just have to take a moment to look.

Our patients have been victims of emotional, sexual, and physical violence. Their ability to trust is limited. When a patient trusts us enough to tell us who they really are, it is a sacred moment. ▼

Keeping Secrets

A nurse remembers the cost—to both patients and herself—of keeping silent about AIDS.

Elena Schwolsky, MPH, RN

In the spring of 1988, two months after my husband, Clarence, was diagnosed with AIDS, I went to work as a pediatric AIDS nurse at a clinic in New Jersey. Clarence had fought in Vietnam, and now he was on the front lines of this epidemic. I felt a need to be there too. It was a time when treatment options ran out fast. The kids I cared for got very sick and soon died. Activists were marching in the streets with signs proclaiming "Silence = Death," but for many, AIDS was something to be whispered about or not spoken of at all. I became a keeper of secrets, and one of them was my own.

"I don't want everyone to see me as your husband who has AIDS, babe," Clarence said. "I want them to know me first as a person, not a disease." I was puzzled—my never-shy husband could get up in a crowded 12-step meeting and declare, "Hi, I'm Clarence and I'm an addict." Why this reluctance? We argued about it, but in the end agreed we'd tell only close friends and family.

Each day I carried my secret to work, where the families I cared for were also hesitant to mention their child's diagnosis. A combination of shame and fear had driven some halfway across the state to avoid being seen in an AIDS clinic in their hometowns. The stigma was intense, even for children, who were considered "innocent" victims. On the nightly news we saw images of a tearful Ryan White, barred from attending school, and a frightened family in Florida burned out of their home. But everyone had their own worries about public disclosure, their own stories to conceal.

There was a child I'll never forget—Jasmine, one of the sickest on my case-load, a bright eight-year-old with a wise little face framed by frizzy brown hair. She lived with her mother and grandmother, but was often in the hospital. I'd usually find her on a comfortably padded stretcher next to the nurses' station.

Concerned that Jasmine might overhear a careless remark on the ward, the social worker and I tried to persuade her mother to tell her that she had AIDS. But Jasmine's mother refused to even discuss it. Perhaps she couldn't bear the guilt over having transmitted the virus to Jasmine. I longed to move beyond the labels that separated us—nurse, wife, mother, person with AIDS—and share my own story. But I kept my promise to Clarence.

One day, as we made rounds, I found Jasmine at her usual post. Pale and listless, with barely enough energy to create another of the crayon drawings that decorated our cubicles, she called me over. "I want to talk to you about something important," she said, obviously making an effort to talk. I prepared myself. Was she going to ask me the question I couldn't answer? Wasn't I bound to respect her mother's wishes?

I leaned over Jasmine's stretcher to hear. "I am very sick," she whispered, pausing for breath. "I think I have AIDS. But you have to promise. Don't tell my mother. It's a secret... She would be sad if she found out."

A few weeks later, at Jasmine's funeral, I wondered if she and her mother had found a way to speak honestly before she died. And again I wished I could have let her mother know how much I shared in her pain.

Clarence died a year later after a long slide, and I no longer had to keep silent. Only then did I begin to acknowledge my own fears. At the bereavement support group, when it was time to share my own story, I "passed," afraid the cancer widows would judge me. For years afterward, when someone would innocently ask, "How did your husband die?" the answer would stick in my throat. I found myself carefully measuring the questioner: Would they ask how he got it?—AIDS always seems to raise that question. And how would they feel about me if they knew?

It's been more than 15 years since I left my job at the clinic. Times have changed and the stigma has diminished. Meanwhile, the incidence of AIDS is on the rise again, particularly among young women of color. I think of the thousands who will be diagnosed this year, and wonder if they will suffer alone, afraid to speak.

The secret I kept for Clarence still has power over me. Even now, when a new acquaintance asks about my late husband, I hesitate. Then I remember Jasmine and that painful silence we all kept back then. I take a breath, and speak in a clear, strong voice: "My husband died of AIDS." ▼

A Man of Few Words

What we don't know about our patients.

Kathryn Mason, MSN, RN, PCCN

Willy had a long last name that we believed to be of Hungarian or Czechoslovakian descent; however, this was purely conjecture. We really didn't know his country of origin, and Willy wasn't talking.

Willy had suffered a debilitating stroke some years earlier and his most striking deficit was profound expressive aphasia. He was unable to articulate more than a few errant words at a time and most of the time his speech consisted of garbled, unintelligible sounds. Willy's affliction belied an otherwise sturdy appearance for a man in his late 70s. He had carved features, with a strong, square chin and gnarled hands that hinted of an earlier life filled with manual labor. I privately imagined that, before his stroke, he had spoken with an accent and a cadence similar to those of Arnold Schwarzenegger.

Our home care agency had maintained Willy on service for several months, treating a nonhealing diabetic wound on his foot. The home health nurses were his only resource: we filled his medication box and made certain that there was food in the house through the Meals on Wheels program (or by bringing food on our visits). The agency provided a home health aide and generally looked after his safety and well-being. It was an unspoken understanding that Willy wouldn't be discharged from services in the near future. We were all willing accomplices.

For a time, I was assigned to be the primary RN on the case. The nursing care plan called for dressing changes to the foot four to five times per week. I made at least three of those visits each week and my routine with Willy became fairly rote. He sat in the same chair each time, with his foot propped on an ottoman; I was positioned in front of the foot, my back to his decrepit television. I would chatter away to compensate for his lack of dialogue, regaling him with stories of my children, the weather, or whatever other bits of news came to mind. Sometimes he would give me his rapt attention and at other times he would be more intent on the news or a game show.

On Labor Day weekend 1997, I found myself unexpectedly having to cover patient visits. It was to have been a holiday off for me and I was annoyed at this sudden change in plans. My family was enjoying a barbecue and company at home while I was traversing rural roads, visiting homebound patients. Like Willy.

Willy was my last visit of the day. When I arrived, he was already ensconced in his chair, awaiting my arrival. He didn't seem to notice my stormy countenance or my marked silence. While I worked on his foot, he continued to watch the news in silence (which somehow irritated me even more). As I neared the end of my task, Willy's foot inexplicably became a squirmy moving target that I was struggling to dress in gauze wrap. Head bent over the foot, determined to swiftly complete the task and head home, I found my attention suddenly arrested by a rich male voice: "The Lady died."

I whipped around to see who had entered the home undetected, but no one was there. Suddenly, I knew—Willy. He had spoken those three words to me, without impediment or hesitation. As I looked incredulously into his face, I realized that he was pointing at the television behind me, where the tragic news of the death of the Princess of Wales had broken into the regularly scheduled program.

On shaking legs, I sank to the ottoman. To this day, I don't know if I was more stunned by the news of Princess Diana or by Willy's unexpected utterance. He was clearly shaken and moved by the death, and I found myself deeply ashamed of my earlier display of petulance. I moved a chair next to his and took his hand. We watched the news of the accident in Paris for about an hour in silence. Willy spoke no more that day, nor did I ever again hear him clearly speak understandable language.

Driving home later that afternoon, it occurred to me that Willy had spoken without a trace of accent, Hungarian or otherwise. ▼

I'm Sorry, Mama

The afternoon of a jail nurse.

Claire Brown, BSN, RN

I called his name, and he stumbled out of the tank of men waiting to be fingerprinted, following me with swaying steps toward my office.

"Please have a seat on the white chair," I said, pointing at a stained plastic seat that quite possibly had been white at one time. Without this directive, inmates usually sat on the short black bench by the door, which was too far from the blood pressure cuff attached to the wall. I pulled out an alcohol assessment form and began.

"I need to ask you some questions about your drinking. I see you already have a chart, so you've been here before. You know the drill."

He smiled at me. The smile of a seasoned drunk is like a baby's guileless and often with the same number of teeth. But this man had all of his. His long black hair was graying, his flat face soft and well boned, and his full lips pretty, almost womanly. But his frame was huge, hulking over the edges of the small chair. His hands, limp in his lap, were dirty, scarred, hard. His eyes were on my hands, filling in his name and date of birth on the form.

"I like your ring," he said. "That's a Navajo piece."

"Thanks, yes it is," I replied. "How long since your last drink?" A standard question, helpful for calculating how long before he would be likely to begin withdrawal—or, in other words, how long I had to process admitting papers, call for doctor's orders, and get him transferred upstairs, safely housed in the infirmary and medicated with Librium before withdrawal seizures began. He didn't reply, so I repeated my question. "How long has it been since you had a drink?"

He raised dark eyes to mine, searched my face for what might be the right answer. Sticky sweet clouds of alcohol and sour sweat surrounded us. Finally he replied, "Well, what time is it?" I attached the blood pressure cuff to his arm and glanced at the clock above his head. "Half past three," I said.

"Three in the morning or three in the afternoon?"

"Three in the afternoon." His blood pressure was 128/84, pulse 76 and regular. He was not nearing detox yet and would probably be fine without Librium for several hours. The nurses upstairs could call for doctor's orders after he'd been moved to the infirmary. Good. One less thing to do. My shift was getting off to a nice slow start.

"Are you sure it's not three in the morning?" he asked.

"Sure I'm sure. I just came in to work. If it were three in the morning, I'd be done already. At home. In bed."

"Then I'm such a bastard." He collapsed forward in the chair, wrapped his arms around his knees and began to cry. "I missed my mother's funeral."

I waited awkwardly, wondering what to say. He made no move to get up. His shoulders were shaking. Finally I asked, "How did she die?"

"She killed herself three days ago in Vancouver. I've been drunk since then. Not that I'm not usually drunk. But I meant to go. I'm sorry, mama. I'm sorry, I'm sorry."

He sat up slowly and began making the sign of the cross in the air. He looked beyond me. "I'm sorry. I'm sorry. Can you ever forgive me? I'm such an asshole." He slumped over again, hugging himself. One arm was still encased in the blood pressure cuff, its stretch cord coiling down from the dial on the wall, disappearing beneath the mass of his plaid flannel back.

"If your mother can hear you, I think she can also see how sad you are. If you were my son, that would matter to me." I was floundering, guessing, hoping that I wasn't going to say the wrong thing and make him angry.

He sat up and stared at me. "You must hate your job," he said.

"No, I don't," I said. "But what makes you say that?"

"You work with criminals all the time."

I paused, trying to fit the word criminal around this softly sad man, charged with public drinking in Pioneer Square. I could see him there, holding the paper bag around the neck of the bottle, finding shelter from the winter rain on the bricks under one of the trees. I said, "Criminals are human beings."

It was the only thing I could think of to say. I could not have told him that I loved my job, that it was never dull, that it provided moments of odd intimacy like this one, that it gave pleasure in knowing what a nurse usually knows—that he or she is almost always of use.

He cried silently a moment more. He said, "That was a good answer." ▼

Convicted

The job description doesn't say you get to choose your patients.

Lisa M. Cook, BS, RN

He was a pedophile, just released from jail after 20 years. His diabetes required two different types of insulin. He had acute renal failure and a recent ileostomy.

"They didn't know what to do with him," the previous nurse said, "so they dumped him on our doorstep." It was now my job, as his patient education nurse, to teach him about diabetes and how to care for the ileostomy.

Before I went into his hospital room, I removed my ID badge and put it in my pocket. I was afraid to let this man know how to locate me or my family. I needed to protect my young daughters.

A frail, toothless old man with straggly gray hair turned to look at me as I introduced myself. He was struggling to move from his bed into a wheelchair. I asked if he needed help.

"No, ma'am," he said. "I can do this. It just takes me a while."

When he was settled in the wheelchair, I asked whether he'd given himself insulin injections and if he had a glucometer.

"They let me check my sugars," he replied, "but I never gave myself a shot." He also said that he took care of emptying and changing his own ileostomy bag.

I pulled up a chair and went over some educational pamphlets with him.

"Wow," he said. "They didn't teach me much in there."

When we finished the session, he thanked me and said he'd read the pamphlets so he could ask questions next time.

As I left, I felt ashamed that I'd taken off my ID badge. After all, I was a nurse, and he wasn't the first ex-convict I'd cared for.

"You really did come back," he said, the next time I visited.

"I told you I would."

"When you're where I was," he said, "you really don't trust people."

He had many good and relevant questions. I taught him how to use a multidose insulin pen. He caught on quickly. Our plan of care was that he would give himself insulin shots with nursing supervision, and I would follow up on his progress.

During my visits over the next two weeks, he would occasionally open up and talk about himself. "I was drinking with my friends and one thing led to another.... I didn't worry about what happened to me while I was in there.... I deserved everything I got.... I ruined a lot of lives with what I did."

Why was he telling me these things? His victim had been a child. I wanted to get away from him. It made me sick to think of the pain and suffering of that child and the family.

On my third or fourth visit he spoke of his childhood, how his father had beaten him. He said he'd joined the army at 15, and still remembered the look on the face of the first person he shot in the Korean War. He had been a POW, and had seen his friend shot after they'd both attempted to escape. He had learned to survive, he said, in "that hole." Once, when he bit down on something hard in the rice they gave him, he realized another tooth had fallen out. Apparently, he'd been traded for, and came back to the United States so malnourished he was almost dead.

"This is no different from prison," he told me, looking around his room. "In fact it's worse. There I could get around and go outside."

This is what I wanted to say, but couldn't: "It was you who made those decisions and acted on them. Whose fault is it that now there's no place for you to go? Who wants a convicted sex offender living next to them?"

One day he told me that social services had found him a place to live and he was leaving. He thanked me for all that I'd done. I told him that I really hadn't done anything special; I was just doing my job. But he insisted that I had. We shook hands. As I walked away, I wished him luck.

"Thanks," he said.

Am I still fearful and disgusted after spending time with a pedophile? Yes, I believe I am. Do I still wonder what I'd do if someone hurt my child? Do I still check the sex offender list to see who's living in my neighborhood? Yes, and yes.

But I did provide nursing care for that patient—a pedophile—as well as I could, just as I'd been taught. Because I'm the one who made the decision to become a nurse, and I don't get to choose those placed in my care. ▼

Edna and the Bedside Tables

Who would pass the test?

Diane M. Goodman, RN

Edna was sharp, all hard edges and bony protrusions. Her face had a ghostly pallor, her hair was thin and limp, and her lips grimaced in disapproval. Although in her mid-seventies and frail, her posture was rigid. She was rarely seen without her robe, which she belted protectively around her emaciated frame. The robe was threadbare, of a faded, indeterminate hue that blended into her skin and made her disappear.

But Edna was anything but invisible. Although hospitalized for severe diverticulitis, she barked demands for coffee and spicy chili during each meal, even as she clutched her abdomen in pain. We'd explained to her that certain foods would exacerbate her intestinal distress, yet she continually blamed her medication. When given pills, she'd dump them on her table, line them up, and question the nurse about each one, an exercise she carried out regularly.

These difficulties were minor compared with the "battles of the bedside table." Edna had two tables, having bribed a technician into bringing an extra one to her room. One table held pens, the nursing call button, eyeglasses, reading material, tissues, and a pair of tattered slippers—all arranged with meticulous order. That wasn't the problem. The issue was with the other table, on which her meals were served.

"No, no, no, you've got it all wrong," Edna would screech as the table was raised and lowered into position. In her eyes, every movement we made was careless. "It has to be one inch from the top of the rail, not over the bed." She demanded that her table be aligned with military precision and that her water glass—neither too full nor too empty—be positioned in exactly the right location. Since the right location changed slightly each meal, the placement of the glass would inevitably result in angry squeals. Soon after she was admitted, the staff began to gather in tense little groups as mealtime approached, whispering and offering one another support. It was as if they were about to draw straws to find out who would serve Edna her meal.

Sue, a patient care technician, was the only staff member who didn't see Edna as a bitter, cantankerous woman. She, instead, saw a woman who rarely received visitors. She saw a woman with sadness in her eyes and a tattered photo of a graying poodle carefully folded among her belongings.

Sue volunteered to bring Edna her meals, determined to pass the test of the table.

"I don't know how you like the table. Perhaps you could show me," Sue offered, the first time she brought Edna her meal. "If I get it wrong, I'll keep trying." For a moment, Edna was quiet, surprised Sue hadn't immediately taken control and pushed the table where she thought it ought to go. Pulling her robe tightly about her shoulders, Edna sat upright, staring at Sue. Sue waited for the tirade, which didn't come. Instead, Edna took her time explaining exactly how she liked things. The table was quietly moved into position and Edna began to eat. It was the same bland food she'd always been served, but this meal was unaccompanied by loud demands for chili.

When I arrived later with Edna's medication, the two women were smiling and talking. Edna took her pills without a quarrel, barely pausing to acknowledge my presence before continuing to share a story with Sue.

The two became allies, as Edna talked about her life. A retired mathematics instructor, she had always been drawn to precision. Yet in the decade since her husband left, her path had become unpredictable and the previous year had been especially difficult. After caring for a younger sister dying of leukemia, her 15-year-old poodle Muffy also died. Childless, she felt alone and afraid. She needed to assert control somewhere and focused on the bedside tables. But once she found companionship through Sue's efforts, the tables lost their importance. She no longer yelled, or even noticed, if they were not perfectly positioned.

Her health improved almost immediately. She began to eat and take her medication without argument; within a few days we discontinued her iv and were looking forward to providing more variety in her diet. She even abandoned the protection of the tattered robe (keeping it neatly folded on her bedside table) and turned on her long-silent television, ready to take interest in the world again.

It took just two bedside tables, one remarkable caregiver, and several measures of compassion to give Edna back her health and her perspective. ▼

Thomas

The safety net catches only those who fall the farthest.

Emily Maloney, BA, EMT-B

Thomas is a frequent flier in our ER, a bespeckled 40-something with coke-bottle glasses, a man who seems to run, like a dog out for a joyride, right into the arms of the dogcatcher. The police bring him in, one man on each arm, his legs limp. Thomas has schizoaffective disorder, dives into the fountain at the mall, screams at strangers at the YMCA, paces outside the grocery store. In a way, I understand—sometimes behaving according to convention can be a little dull.

Thomas always comes into our ER in the same way, accompanied to one of our dedicated psychiatric rooms. They're easy to strip and you can lock the cabinets with a key affixed by a strong magnet to the Pyxis at the nursing station. This is a tech's job: to strip the room after getting him vitaled and find a plastic bag for his clothes. I wear gloves. He's stopped taking his Seroquel, was picked up for hassling customers outside a Life Time Fitness franchise.

"*Listen*," Thomas says, irritated that he's with us again.

"Yes, Thomas?" I stuff his clothes into the bag. When it's not a psych patient, I usually fold them—patients complain. Besides, they're filthy.

"I need," he says, exasperated, "a *sandwich*!"

We look each other in the eye, hard. In some ways, his life seems easier than mine: I'm working at this hospital so that I'll be covered under a group health insurance policy that allows me—for about $100 a month plus copays—to see my psychiatrist, 232 miles away. I've tried to find someone closer to home, but so far no one seems right. (Later, it will turn out that my complaint is medical rather than psychiatric, but for now, I go with it.)

Thomas has no job, no worry of an ability to pay for service rendered. There is no question of financial insolvency—here he is, a ward of the state, resplendent in two gowns, one forward, one backward to cover the gap. And he wants a sandwich.

I look up at the ER board. His nurse is Sara. Across the ER, Sara holds a kidney basin to the chin of her patient, an elderly woman, who pukes into it. A practical person, a graduate of a diploma nursing program, Sara's trying life in the big city. I ask her if I can get Thomas a sandwich.

"Sure," she says. I go to get the sandwich. One of the other techs sits outside the psych room, keeping an eye on Thomas.

Hours later, when Thomas is admitted, I accompany him to his room. He has some kind of heart problem, a little gallop, maybe an electrical issue, which is why they send him to a monitoring floor instead of the psych ward. But they need a sitter, a body to stay in his room all night. They're short on float pool nurses and Mary, one of the ER nurses, has volunteered me. Built like a washing machine or maybe a narwhal, she disimpacts 98-year-old dementia patients with ease, throws iv pumps at unsuspecting techs. I'm afraid of her, which is why I say OK. Plus there's overtime at stake.

But it's a bad idea—I need sleep to metabolize the medications I don't need.

When they set us up on 3-West, I worry: 3-West is known for strange lapses in care, for people coding in the middle of the night, gasping for air or water like antediluvian animals. None of the rooms are really private, which means we share ours with an empty bed on the other side of the curtain. I find a chair and settle in.

Tomorrow, Thomas will be released to the adult psychiatry ward, which will release him back outside. His sleep apnea will persist, and those small Seroquel tablets pressed into his palm before bed will disappear from his system just 18 hours after he leaves our little community hospital. There are other ways of administering the Seroquel so he'd only have to show up at his group home or community service agency once a week or even twice a month. Still …

He shudders in his sleep. He's 43 years old, and in this dark room, illuminated only by a strip of incandescent light from the parking lot, he mumbles softly, like a child. I'm exhausted. When the traveling nurse comes to relieve me in the morning, I mumble incoherently. Thomas sleeps on, fueled by the Seroquel. I stumble out into the harsh morning light, struggle to find my car, and drive home to my apartment, where I examine my medications before taking them, two little eyes, staring up at me: chalky pills in my palm. ▼

References

The following are the original citations of the essays reprinted in this book. The *American Journal of Nursing (AJN)* is grateful to the authors for their permission.

All in the Family

Lois A. Gerber, MPH, RN. "Two Nurses – One Old, One New," AJN 2010;110(7):72

Peggy Vincent, RN, CNM. "Morphine. Now.," AJN 2002;102(2):25

Karen Schoonmaker, MSN, RN, CNL. "At the Eye of the Storm," AJN 2012;112(9):72

Elizabeth Corso Falter, RN, CNAA, BC. "Census of One, Staff of Five," AJN 2002;102(4):25

Donna Diers, PhD, RN, FAAN. "A Nurse's Mother's Nurses," AJN 2008;108(2):88

Carrie A. Bennett, MS, CNS-BC. "A Place for Palliative Care," AJN 2010;110(4):72

Career Is a Forking Path

Cortney Davis, MA, RN, ANP. "The Fine Art," AJN 2008;108(5):52

Meredith Bailey, MSN, BSN, RN, PMH-NP. "Making it Fit," AJN 2014;114(6):72

John B. Fiddler, MSN, RN, ACHPN. "Intensive Care," AJN 2014;114(5):72

Donna Diers, PhD, RN, FAAN. "Am I A Nurse?," AJN 2005;105(10):39

Cheryl Dellasega, PhD, CRNP. "A Moment of Grace," AJN 2005;105(2):39

Judy Morse, ASN, RN. "Promises to Keep," AJN 2006;106(7):39

Beverly Rossiter, MSN, CRNP, CPNP. "The Eyes of a Pediatric Nurse," AJN 2006;106(2):39

Colleagues, for Better or Worse

Evelyn Lawson-Jonsson, BSN, RN. "Roger's Angst," AJN 2011;111(4):72

Natosha Cramer, BSN, RN. "The Blame Game," AJN 2014;114(4):72

Nancy L. Ball, RN. "Who's the Fool?," AJN 2008;108(12):88

Cindy McCoy, PhD, MSN, RN-BC. "Ordinary Things," AJN 2007;107(12):88

Corina DeVries, RN. "Deception," AJN 2004;104(2):39

Doctor Jekyll and Doctor Hyde

John A. Forrant, BSN, RN, CCRN. "Last Rights," AJN 2008;108(8):88

Michael M. Bloomfield, MD. "My Turn," AJN 2015;115(12):72

Ann Fleming Beach, MD. "A Smart Doctor Listens to the Nurses," AJN 2013;113(4):72

From the Other Side

Jennifer K. Englund, MSEd. "Seized," AJN 2012;112(6):72

Tiana Tozer. "The Brat," AJN 2013;113(12):70

Susan Luton. "The Game of What If?," AJN 2008;108(3):88

Andrew Merton. "The Third Way," AJN 2008;108(10):88

Amy Noel Green. "Every Three Months," AJN 2013;113(9):72

Joy Ladin. "Intake Interview," AJN 2009;109(7):72

Gail Lukasik, MA, PhD. "A Passing Shadow," AJN 2011;111(12):72

Tim Bascom. "A Stone of Contention," AJN 2010;110(2):72

Susan Clements. "Swabbing Tubby," AJN 2015;115(2):72

Sandra Stone. "To the Child They Were All One Kind," AJN 2006;106(11):88

Linda Meierhoffer, MS, MPA, BA. "Breathing Room," AJN 2008;108(6):88

Getting Started

Ray Bingham, RNC, "The Prospering of Cheaters," AJN 2001;101(4):45

Sally Bellerose, RN. "Touchy-Feely Stuff," AJN 2002;102(7):25

Lyssa Friedman, RN, BSN, MPA. "Where's My Hospice Moment?," AJN 2001;101(11):25

Judith L. Reishtein, PhD, RN. "My First Preceptor," AJN 2014;114(3):72

Kathleen Hughes, MSN, RN, PNP-BC. "Bed Bath," AJN 2014;114(1):72

Elizabeth Tillotson, BS. "A Nurse? What Was I Thinking?," AJN 2012;112(11):72

Janet L. Richards, BSN, RN. "A Special Kind of Knowledge," AJN 2013;113(1):72

Nancy Walters, RN. "Coming Home to Nursing," AJN 2015;115(9):72

Heartbreakers
Cheryl A. Dellasega, PhD, RN, CRNP. "The Grief Train," AJN 2013;113(10):72

Amanda L. Richmond, BSN, RN-BC. "The Hardest Decision," AJN 2013;113(2):72

V. Jude Forbes, MSN, FNP. "The Price of a Miracle," AJN 2005;105(3):38

Arlene Koch, RN. "No Regrets," AJN 2003;103(5):31

Lorraine Randall, RNC. "Florida Vacation," AJN 2003;103(3):31

Sam Bastian, MS, ARPN, BC. "In the Hand of Dad," AJN 2002;102(8):43

Dawne De Voe Olbrych, MSN, RN, CNS. "Inseparable," AJN 2002;102(12):25

Karen Rousch, MSN, RN, FNP. "Steven," AJN 2006;106(3):39

Lessons Learned
Kathleen L. Sitzman, MS, RN. "The Ice-Bag Incident," AJN 2004;104(7):39

Maureen Anthony, MSN, RN, CS, CDE. "Nurse, Heal Thyself," AJN 2004;104(3):39

Cortney Davis, MA, NP, RN. "The Pain," AJN 2006;106(10):88

Meg Sniderman, RN. "At the Night Camp," AJN 2010;110(12):72

Shixiang Luo, MSN, RN. "Skipped Two Times," AJN 2013;113(3):72

Dorothy Miller, RN. "Tending Mr. Brown," AJN 2006;106(12):88

Making A Difference
Danielle Allen, RN. "Am I Going to Be Okay?," AJN 2015;115(3):72

Bryanne Hickey Harrington, BSN, RN, CNOR. "Socks and All…," AJN 2011;111(1):72

Nancy Cabianca, RN. "A Change of Heart," AJN 2014;114(12):72

Kelly Carroll, BA, RN. "A Brief Respite," AJN 2004;104(8):39

Marie F. Kerscher, Bed, RN (Coordinated by Veneta Masson, MA, RN). "May I Have a Band-Aid?," AJN 2001;101(9):25

Alice C. Facente, MSN, RN, BC. "The Dirtiest House in Town," AJN 2010;110(1):72

Susan L. Goff, MS, RN. "What One Thing Will Make Today Better for You?," AJN 2011;111(9):72

Memorable Patients
Cheryl Kane, Med, BSN, RN. "Hiding a Tender Soul," AJN 2013;113(12):72

Elena Schwolsky, MPH, RN. "Keeping Secrets," AJN 2011;111(10):72

Kathryn Mason, MSN, RN, PCCN. "A Man of Few Words," AJN 2012;112(8):72

Claire Bowen, BSN, RN. "I'm Sorry, Mama," AJN 2006;106(5):39

Lisa M. Cook, BS, RN. "Convicted," AJN 2010;110(3):72

Diane M. Goodman, RN. "Edna and the Bedside Tables," AJN 2003;103(12):31

Emily Maloney, BA, EMT-B. "Thomas," AJN 2013;113(7):72

Navigating the System
Robbie Ravert, RN, RNC-OB. "Before the Signal Fades," AJN 2011;111(7):72

Joyce Hislop, RN, OCN. "Paper Chart Nurse," AJN 2010;110(10):72

Cynthia Stock, MSN, RN, CCRN. "Final Connection," AJN 2015;115(11):72

Lorraine Dale, RN. "Chaos," AJN 2002;102(10):25

Marie E. Lasater, MSN, RN, CCRN, CNRN. "Heads and Beds," AJN 2008;108(11):88

Tables Turned
Joan Schmidt, MS-MPH, RN, ACRN. "To Mania and Back," AJN 2004;104(6):31

Alice C. Facente, MSN, RN-BC. "At Her Mercy," AJN 2009;109(8):72

Marcia Gardner, MA, RN, CRNP, CPN. "Big Love," AJN 2004;104(9):39

Jean DiMotto, JD, MSN, RN. "A Mind in Search of Its Moorings," AJN 2013;113(12):71

Suellen Hozman, BS, RN. "The Other Cancer Story," AJN 2005;105(11):39

Marilyn Wargo, BSN, RNC. "The Enduring Self," AJN 2006;106(6):39

Madeleine Mysko, MA, RN. "The Sacraments of Sister Thecla," AJN 2011;111(5):72